Self-Harm in Young People

Dennis Ougrin & Sum Yu Pansy Yue

Published by iConcept Press Limited

Published by iConcept Press Limited

Copyright © iConcept Press 2016

http://www.iconceptpress.com

ISBN: 978-1-922227-17-1

First published 2016. Reprinted 2016 (with corrections).

Printed in the United States of America

Contents

Preface

Self-harm in adolescents is a growing problem which has been poorly defined, clinically neglected and insufficiently researched. This volume synthesizes the available research on adolescent self-harm and presents the reader with the best available evidence on self-harm treatment. It is aimed at those who treat, research and teach about self-harm.

1

Defining Self-Harm

Without a clear definition at the beginning, it is impossible to interpret any literature on self-harm. Despite the fact that self-harm in humans has existed for millennia across various cultures and geographical locations (1), controversy remains to this day about the definitions and nomenclature used regarding self-harm.

1.1   The Historical Divide in Defining Self-Harm

Since 1938, there have been attempts at categorising suicide-related and self-mutilative behaviour (2). It was Kreitman's seminal work in 1969 on parasuicide (3) that led to the broadly defined concepts behind the contemporary definitions of suicidal behaviour used across Europe today (4, 5). Kreitman's broadly defined concepts contrast with the contemporary American perspective based on the work of Beck and colleagues (6, 7). Unlike Kreitman's concepts, the American perspective views intent as key in classifying suicidal behavior. This historical divide remains to this day, between those who believe that self-harm should be categorised into that with and without intent to die, and those who believe that self-harm should represent a broad spectrum of self-harmful behaviour irrespective of suicidal intent. We will arbitrarily refer to the former, predominantly American approach as the "Beck-O'Carroll-Silverman" nomenclature and the latter, predominantly European/Australasian approach as the "Kreitman-Hawton-De Leo" nomenclature.

1.2   Self-Harm Nomenclature

It is important to note that nomenclature and classification are distinct terms. Whilst nomenclature revolves around terminology and definitions to define basic concepts, classification seeks to describe the relevant phenomena, which can only be done with clear nomenclature. Self-harm nomenclature is generally based on four concepts: intent, method, outcome and lethality.

1.3   What is Intent?

Intent can be defined as the objective that you plan to achieve: an aim or purpose (8). It is similar but distinct from motivation (9), the driving force behind intent. Differentiating between subjective and objective intent is difficult (10), and controversy surrounds the role of intent in the definition of self-harm. Many also believe that intent is hard to measure reliably, as a plethora of reasons often exist for self-harm (4, 11) and some so-called suicide attempts have been shown to be self-harm without suicidal intent (12). To measure intent, Beck *et al.* developed the Suicide Intent Scale (SIS) in 1974 (7). A similar scale was also subsequently designed by Pierce *et al.* (13). Even though some evidence suggests that the Beck SIS is not a strong predictor for identifying individuals who would ultimately die of suicide (14), the importance of assessing intent as part of risk assessments and as a guide for clinical management is generally accepted. More recently, Posner *et al.* (15) developed the Columbia Classification Algorithm of Suicide Assessment (C-CASA), designed to differentiate between suicidal and non-suicidal self-harm. C-CASA has been shown to provide reliable ratings and it offers a distinct advantage of including a category for indeterminate events where suicidal intent is unknown (15).

1.4   What are Lethality, Outcome and Method?

Lethality can be defined as danger to life (16). It represents the potential for death given the means used for self-harm (17). Objective lethality has clearly been associated with the risk of dying by suicide (18) and with suicidal intent (19). However, about a third of near-fatal self-harm cases report no suicidal intent (20). For example, Brown *et al.* found minimal association between suicide intent and medical lethality for attempted suicides (21). This suggests that perhaps suicidal intent and lethality are distinct aspects of suicidal behaviour. Notably, half of the subjects in the study had inaccurate expectations of the actual lethality of their attempt. It has therefore been suggested that subjective lethality may be a better predictor of risk than objective lethality. In any case, evidence suggests that the relationships between lethality, intent and future suicidal behavior are complex (19) and not very well understood to date. None-the-less, clinically both objective and subjective lethality need to be evaluated.

Method can be described as the process used by the subject to self-harm, leading to possible outcomes: death or survival with or without injuries. A variety of methods are used for self-harm, and some authors use method as a way of defining research populations, for example those who have taken an overdose of medication or those who have injured themselves by cutting (22 – 24), avoiding the need to use definitions based on more subjective measures.

1.5   The "Beck-O'Carroll-Silverman" Nomenclature

The Beck-O'Carroll-Silverman nomenclature divides suicide-related behaviours into instrumental suicide-related behaviour with no intent to die, and suicidal acts with intent to die. Relatively recently, this nomenclature was revised (25), proposing that intent could also be undetermined and that subjects could have sustained no or some injuries, or may even have died as a result. This was a welcome acknowledgement of the European approach of defining self-harm irrespective of suicidal intent and the fact that "deliberate self-harm" has been largely replaced with the term "self-harm" in Europe. However, this revision still has flaws, having not accounted for lethality or the issue of suicide-related communication and thinking without suicidal intent.

1.6   The "Kreitman-Hawton-De Leo" Nomenclature

Based on Kreitman's original definition of parasuicide, Hawton et al. (26) defined self-harm as intentional self-injury or self-poisoning, irrespective of motivation or suicidal intent. More recently, De Leo et al. (27) noted the evolution of their definition of self-harm over the years as they conducted their WHO/EURO study. Initially, their definition was quite similar to that used in the UK today, but eventually introduced an outcome-based approach, using "fatal" and "non-fatal" to describe suicidal-behaviour (27). The role of intent in non-fatal suicidal behaviour remained ambiguous and the authors acknowledged that even collaborators of the same big trial may disagree and alter their definitions over time. Limitations of the Kreitman-Hawton-De Leo approach include the focus on self-harm as a behaviour, neglecting suicidal or self-harm thinking, as well as largely disregarding lethality and suicidal intent.

1.7   Characteristics That May Help Categorise Self-Harm

Since intent is not easily and reliably measured, researchers have investigated whether other characteristics ranging from co-morbidities to clinical features may help differentiate between suicidal and non-suicidal self-harm.

Psychiatric and personality disorders are common in suicidal and non-suicidal self-harm patients. In a study of a representative sample of 150 self-harm patients, 92% met the diagnostic criteria for psychiatric disorders, with depression being the most common (28). Nearly half (45.9%) of the participants in the same study had personality disorders. This study was not limited to adolescents but limited to patients who presented to a general hospital, who may have higher prevalence rates of co-morbid psychiatric or personality disorders than that found in the general adolescent population. The researchers of the study acknowledged that there may have been some bias towards subjects with greater psychopathology because not all potential subjects could be included in the study (28). Despite the limitations, it is clear that self-harm patients may frequently have co-morbid psychiatric or personality disorders, which require assessment and management alongside any care they receive for self-harm.

Negative life events and life problems are also common in those who self-harm, with one large study finding 80.6% of self-harm patients presenting to hospital reported multiple life problems, most commonly regarding interpersonal relationships (29). A weak positive correlation was found in the same study between the number of life problems and suicidal intent in females (but not males) with no past history of self-harm. This finding was similarly noted in a separate study by Crane and colleagues

(30), suggesting that self-harm patients with high suicidal intent presenting with no past history of self-harm may be experiencing a somewhat different set of life problems than those with low suicidal intent (30).

A host of other factors, including impulsivity, engagement in health
risk behaviours and being in a single-parent family, have been suggested
to help differentiate those who engage in non-suicidal self-harm versus
those who engage in suicidal self-harm (31). In addition, adolescents with
suicidal self-harm may have a later age of onset of self-harm, use self-
poisoning more often than self-injury and may respond less well to psychological interventions than adolescents with non-suicidal self-harm (32).
Adolescents who engage in non-suicidal self-harm may have fewer depressive symptoms, greater parental support and self-esteem (33) than the
one who self-harm with suicidal intent.

In addition, there is evidence for a genetic basis for self-harm, which
will be discussed in greater detail in Chapter 3. Several studies have found
neurobiological or physiological differences in people whom self-harm as
well; they will be reviewed in more detail in Chapter 4.

1.8   Non-Suicidal Self-Injury (NSSI)

One particular type of self-harm called "Non-Suicidal Self-Injury" (NSSI)
has been emerging as a distinct sub-category. It can be defined as the "direct, deliberate destruction of one's own body tissue in the absence of intent to die" (34). Its prev-
alence in adolescents worldwide is estimated to be in the range of 10-40%
(35).

NSSI is strongly associated with suicide attempts (36, 37), and the
two behaviours often co-occur, with an increase in one behaviour associated with an increase in the other (38). In fact, in depressed adolescents, a
history of NSSI behaviour may be an even stronger predictor of future suicide attempts than recent suicide attempts (37, 39).

Whilst strong associations between NSSI and suicidal self-harm exist, NSSI is distinct from suicidal behaviour in several key ways. NSSI can
typically be differentiated by its intent, lethality and repetition. By definition, unlike those who engage in suicidal self-injury, individuals who engage in NSSI do not have the intent to die nor do they believe that they
will die from their NSSI behaviour (40). Whereas suicidal self-harm is of-

ten characterised by high lethality, low frequency behaviour, NSSI differs with its typically low lethality, high frequency, repetitive self-injurious behaviour (38). Although the use of dangerous methods of self-harm may indicate higher suicidal intent, the method used is not a reliable indicator of intent and all individuals who present with self-harm, irrespective of method, should receive psychosocial assessment (41).

The term "NSSI" has certain limitations. Using "non-suicidal" may be viewed as misleading, given the strong association between NSSI and suicidal behaviour. Suicidal intent is also often ambiguous, leading to difficulty in separating NSSI and suicide attempts. A third limitation of NSSI is that by definition, it does not include self-poisoning or overdoses, even when patients clearly report that there was no intent to die. Nevertheless, as evidence continues to emerge separating NSSI from suicide attempts, NSSI has recently been recognised as an independent condition in the Diagnostic and Statistical Manual of Mental Disorders, Fifth Edition (42). It is hoped that its inclusion, albeit with the proviso of further research to be undertaken, would stimulate this field of enquiry (43).

1.9   Conclusion: Self-Harm – A Broad Spectrum of Behaviour

In summary, self-harm can be seen as a spectrum of behaviours, encompassed by the broad definition of self-poisoning or self-injury irrespective of suicidal intent. For clarity, we will state whether the results of the studies reviewed in this book apply to adolescents with self-harm, suicide attempts, or NSSI where these distinctions are clear. When we refer to "self-harm," we are referring to the broad definition used in the United Kingdom and Europe that includes NSSI, suicide attempts, and self-harm with undetermined intent.

2

The Prevalence and Natural History of Self-Harm

Determining the prevalence of self-harm presents researchers with a considerable challenge. It is highly dependent on a range of factors, including the definition of self-harm used, the detection tools, survey type, timeframe covered, as well as the age of the participants and population studied. This has led to a range of prevalence figures reported in literature. In a systematic review of the international prevalence of self-harm in adolescents worldwide, lifetime prevalence of self-harm in community samples of adolescents reportedly ranged from 2.9 to 42% (35), whereas the lifetime prevalence of self-harm in hospitalized adolescent has been reported as high as 82% (44).

2.1   Detection Tools Used

The wide range of different detection tools used in self-harm research limits our ability to compare and collate prevalence data from different studies. The lack of a universal, gold standard self-harm detection tool or a consensus on which tools are the most accurate represent major challenges in establishing the true prevalence of self-harm in adolescents. Here we present a brief overview of some examples of those tools, presented in Table 2.1.

Structured and semi-structured diagnostic interviews are commonly used in studies, which are typically small in size for practical reasons. The wording of questions designed to assess self-harm varies greatly between the different tools. Although the time period covered by different interview-based methods usually differ, most tend to cover the entire lifetime by using phrases such as "have you ever…" in their questions. There are also differences in the range of behaviours assessed, the thresholds for which the behaviours are identified as present. A comparison of the Child and Adolescent Psychiatric Assessment (CAPA) with the Diagnostic Interview for Children and Adolescents (DICA) tools is presented in Table 2.2.

Interview-Based Diagnostic Tools	Self-Report Questionnaires	Functional Assessment
Child and Adolescent Psychiatric Assessment (CAPA) (45)	Deliberate Self-Harm Inventory (DSHI) (46)	Functional Assessment of Self-Mutilation (FASM) (47)
Diagnostic Interview for Children and Adolescents (DICA) (48)	Self-Harm Behaviour Questionnaire (SHBQ) (49)	
The Kiddie-Schedule for Affective Disorders and Schizophrenia Present and Lifetime Version (K-SADS-PL) (50)	Self-Harm Questionnaire (SHQ) (51)	
	Self-Harm Inventory (SHI) (52)	

Table 2.1: Examples of Detection Tools Used to Assess Self-Harm Prevalence.

	The CAPA (45)	The DICA (48)
Age Group Covered (Years Old)	9 – 17	6 – 17
Range of Disorders Covered	DSM-III, DSM-IV, ICD-10	DSM-III, DSM-IV, ICD-10
Requirements of Interviewer	At Least Bachelor-level degree	Lay but highly trained
Specifically Identifies Suicidal Ideation	Yes	Yes
Specifically Identifies Suicidal Self-Harm	Yes	Yes
Specifically Identifies Non-Suicidal Self-Harm	Yes	No

Table 2.2: Comparing the Child and Adolescent Psychiatric Assessment (CAPA) with the Diagnostic Interview for Children and Adolescents (DICA).

Although the CAPA and the DICA cover slightly different age rang-es, they do cover a similar, broad range of conditions (45, 48). While both the CAPA and DICA include questions designed to identify suicidal self-harm and suicidal ideation, a significant difference between the two is that only the CAPA includes questions directed at identifying non-suicidal self-harm. The K-SADS-PL is another tool that also assesses non-suicidal self-harm, as well as suicidal ideation and suicide attempts (53).

On the other hand, there are many types of self-report question-naires available for self-harm detection and assessment. They tend to in-herently be easier to administer, so are more likely to be used in studies with a relatively larger sample size than those employing interview-based methods. The DSHI and the SHBQ were developed over a decade ago and have been shown to be relatively reliable (54). The SHQ (51) is primarily a screening tool improving detection rate of self-harm compared with usual psychiatric assessment. The SHQ also includes questions directed at iden-tifying the emotions surround the most recent self-harm episode, if one exists, and identifying the self-reported intent for that episode (51).

Finally, another approach to assessing self-harm prevalence is via a functional assessment of self-harm. The Functional Assessment of Self-Mutilation (FASM) is an example of such a tool, which has also been found to be relatively reliable (47). The FASM covers a wider range of behaviours (e.g. picking of wounds) than some of the other assessment tools and the prevalence rate reported using the FASM is often higher than with other tools.

It is not just the wording of the detection tool itself that can influence self-harm prevalence findings. Other factors such as the setting in which the self-harm assessment is made (55) and whether it is the adolescents or their parents that are the key source of information (56) are important too.

2.2   Prevalence of Self-Harm

To date, the most comprehensive review of self-harm prevalence in ado-lescents included collating 128 studies with a total of 513,188 adolescents (57). Although this review of self-harm literature worldwide was done a decade ago, it has several key strengths, including the fact that it did not limit the studies collected by language and collated prevalence data for different types of self-harm. From the review, 9.7% (95% CI, 8.5 – 10.9) of adolescents on average reported having attempted suicide in their lifetime, of which 6.4% (95% CI, 5.4 – 7.5) occurred in the previous year. The mean proportion of adolescents who engaged in self-harm in their lifetime was 13.2% (95%CI, 8.1 – 18.3). A mean of 29.9% (95% CI, 26.1 – 33.8) of adolescents reported having had suicidal thoughts at some point in their lives, 19.3% (95%CI, 11.7 – 27.0) having had such thoughts in the previous year. The review also highlighted a significantly higher prevalence of both suicidal thoughts and behaviours in females compared to males, and this was supported by the results of 88 out of 128 studies that reported prevalence separately for males and females (57). Epidemiological evidence suggests that males are more likely than females to use highly lethal methods of self-harm (58) and since numerous studies rely on data from hospital presentations of self-harm, it may be that the prevalence of self-harm in females is underestimated in such studies, making the gender difference even more striking.

In addition, the review found significant within-group variation beyond that expected by chance in adolescents who reported suicidal thoughts and attempts; for example for those reporting lifetime suicidal thoughts, the prevalence reported varied from 8% to 70%. It is believed that this variation most likely reflects differences in study methodology and the cohort populations studied. This is supported by other findings of the review, where studies that used anonymous questionnaires generally reported higher prevalence figures of suicidal behaviour versus those that used interview-based assessments. Self-harm prevalence figures in the previous 6 months and suicidal thoughts in the previous year were also higher for studies using anonymous versus non-anonymous questionnaires, with the difference being statistically significant (57).

Since the publication of this review, other studies have also attempted to establish the prevalence of self-harm in adolescents. Muehlenkamp and colleagues (35) differentiated between non-suicidal self-injury (NSSI) and deliberate self-harm (DSH) prevalence rates, acknowledging the different definitions of the two terms. A mean lifetime prevalence of 18.0% (SD = 7.3) and 16.1% (SD = 11.6) for NSSI and DSH was observed, with a statistically insignificant difference between the two. The review noted that the range of methodologies and assessment tools used contributed much to the variation in self-harm prevalence between studies, with assessments that involved single-item questions tending to report lower prevalence rates than those that involved specific behaviour checklists. The difference between the two assessment modalities for DSH studies was statistically significant, suggesting that the type of assessment tool used in studies may be a potential source of bias.

Another notable study conducted since 2005 is the Child & Adolescent Self-Harm in Europe (CASE) Study (59). Spanning seven countries, this large multi-centre investigation included over 30, 000 adolescents (mainly 15 – 16 year olds) in schools across Australia, England, Ireland, Hungary, Belgium, the Netherlands and Norway. Using the Lifestyle and Coping Questionnaire, the CASE Study observed a mean lifetime prevalence of self-harm (at least one episode fitting strict criteria based on Hawton's definition of self-harm discussed in Chapter 1) in females and males of 13.5% and 4.3% respectively. 8.9% of females and 2.6% of males reported such an episode in the previous year. International differences in the prevalence of self-harm were observed as well, ranging from 3.6% in the Netherlands to 11.8% in Australia for females and from 1.7% in the Netherlands and Hungary to 4.3% in Belgium for males.

The most commonly reported reason for self-harm in that study was "to get relief from a terrible state of mind", with the second most common reason being "to die". Reporting multiple reasons for an episode of self-harm was common, especially in females (88%) relative to males (72.6%). There appeared to be some relationship between the method used for self-harm and a few of the possible 8 reasons given for that episode of self-harm. For females, the reason "I wanted to punish myself" was most strongly associated with self-cutting only (52.3%), other single methods (46.6%), but less so for multiple methods (36.8%) and overdose only (30.5%). For males, the reason "I wanted to find out whether someone really loved me" was most commonly given for overdose only (42.6%) and multiple methods (41.9%) rather than single methods or self-cutting only (both 26.2%). More recent analysis of the findings of the CASE Study identified female gender, high impulsivity, history of physical or sexual abuse, concerns about sexual orientation and experience of self-harm or suicide of others as independent factors that differentiated those who only had self-harm thoughts versus those who actually engaged in an episode of self-harm (60). In addition, the analysis identified other factors such as depression, anxiety, impulsivity and lower self-esteem that were associated with self-harm history of greater severity.

A third notable study that reported prevalence rates of self-harm in adolescents is the Saving and Empowering Young Lives in Europe (SEYLE) intervention study (61). This large, multi-centre, cluster-randomised controlled trial was conducted in randomly selected schools in 11 European countries (Austria, Estonia, France, Germany, Hungary, Ireland, Israel, Italy, Romania, Slovenia and Spain) and recruited a considerable total sample size of 12, 395 adolescents (median age being 15 years old) at baseline (62). The prevalence of risky behaviours (including excessive alcohol use, sedentary behaviour, high use of internet/TV/video games unrelated to school or work, being underweight) was assessed, allowing the use of latent class analysis to separate the large adolescent cohort into three groups (low-risk, high-risk, invisible risk) depending on how frequently they engaged in those risky behaviours. Adolescents were classed as part of the "invisible risk" group if they scored highly for use of internet/TV/video games unrelated to school or work, sedentary behaviour and reduced sleep. Whilst the prevalence of suicidal thoughts in the "invisible risk" group was found to be comparable to that in the "high-risk" group (42.4% vs. 44%), the prevalence of suicide attempts in the "high-risk" group was 10.1%, almost twice that of the 5.9% in the "invisible risk" group (63). The reason for this disparity is unclear, although it may be that those in the "invisible risk" group are more likely to internalize their emotions or thoughts and less likely to act on them than those in the "high-risk" groups. This is reflected in the prevalence of NSSI in the three groups, being 5.5%, 12.4% and 22.3% for the low-risk, invisible-risk and high-risk groups respectively.

2.3   Prevalence of NSSI in Adolescents

The field of non-suicidal self-injury (NSSI) research in adolescents is relatively new, with most studies only conducted in the past decade or so. NSSI assessment tools have traditionally been limited to non-specific tools part of suicide assessments or tools that only assess a limited range of NSSI characteristics (64). In fact, only very recently has a NSSI-specific assessment tool (called the Non-Suicidal Self-Injury-Assessment Tool or NSSI-AT) been developed and preliminarily validated for its reliability (64).

The latest review in this area estimated that internationally, the prevalence of NSSI in adolescents is in the ranges of 15 – 46% in the community and 40 – 80% in clinical populations (65). The ranges reflect significant variation between studies. In a previous systematic review, the mean NSSI prevalence in adolescents from international studies from 2005 to 2011 was calculated to be 18.0% with a relatively large standard deviation of 7.3% (35). The few existing older studies from the 1990s on NSSI prevalence in adolescents have generally found lower prevalence rates than more recent studies conducted during the past 10 – 15 years. Whether this observation is due to changes in methodology over time or reflects true changes in NSSI prevalence in adolescent populations over time is unclear, although the huge difference in the prevalence estimates between the older and the newer studies makes differences in reporting an unlikely explanation. For example, a study conducted in 1993 found the prevalence of NSSI to be 2.46% for males and 2.79% for females (66). Another study conducted in 1997 estimated 12-month NSSI prevalence in a sample of Australian adolescents to be 4.9% (67). These two studies contrast sharply with for example, one cross-national study in 2012 that observed a mean NSSI prevalence of 24% in the previous year after adjusting for socio-demographic variation (68). Another recent study found the yearly NSSI prevalence estimate to be 10.01% in a sample of 1,582 Flemish adolescents (69). For lifetime prevalence rates, studies have found rates to range from 13.71% in Flemish adolescents (69) to 52.7% in adolescent offspring of male Croatian combat-related post-traumatic stress disorder (PTSD) veterans (70).

Some studies have found a significant gender difference in NSSI prevalence, suggesting that perhaps NSSI is more prevalent in females than males. Evidence in this area is conflicting. For example, age-standardised prevalence rates of NSSI have been shown to be 6.3% higher in females than males in one study (71), whilst another study found comparable lifetime NSSI prevalence rates (49.4% in females vs. 48% in males) between the two genders (72). In a recent meta-analysis (73) NSSI prevalence was generally 1.5 times higher in women than men (26.36% in men vs. 33.78% in women, OR = 1.5, 95%CI = 1.35, 1.65, p < 0.001). Significant heterogeneity in effect size across the studies included in the meta-analysis was also noted. In addition, studies that used interview-based assessment tools tended to observe larger gender differences than those that used self-reporting assessment tools.

Another observation of note is that NSSI remains relatively common in high-functioning adolescent populations with one study in 2,875 American university students reporting prevalence rates of approximately 25% (74). NSSI is also prevalent amongst socioeconomically privileged youths. Evidence suggests that NSSI rates may be as high as 37.2% in this class of adolescents, with parental criticism being a factor associated with increased NSSI (75).

2.4   Hospital Presentations of Self-Harm in Adolescents

Although it is known that episodes of self-harm that present in hospitals differ in some ways (e.g. self-poisoning overdoses are more likely to present in hospital compared to self-cutting) from episodes that occur in the community, hospital presentations of self-harm represent an important and often used source of data for studies on self-harm prevalence.

The most comprehensive source of data regarding self-harm presentations in hospital in the United States is from the National Center for Injury Prevention and Control as part of the Centers for Disease Control and Prevention (CDC). Unlike the definitions of self-harm typically used in America (Chapter 1), the CDC's definition of self-harm does not differentiate between suicidal and non-suicidal self-harm, instead including suicides, suicide attempts and other intentional self-harm (76). This source of data comprises all self-harm presentations to emergency departments in hospitals across the United States and is easily accessible online via the Web-based Injury Statistics Query and Reporting System (WISQARS) on the National Center for Injury Prevention and Control's website. From the WISQARS non-fatal injury report, self-harm presentations in those aged 1 – 18 increased significantly from 89.21 per 100,000 in 2001 to 138.22 per 100,000 in 2013 (77). One of the most striking observations from this data is that females in this age group are consistently two to three times more likely to present to hospital with self-harm every year.

A similarly comprehensive but smaller source of data regarding hospital presentations of self-harm in the United Kingdom (UK) is the Oxford Monitoring System for Attempted Suicide. Since 1976, it has registered hospital presentations of self-harm in Oxford annually. Like the CDC, the definition of self-harm used is one irrespective of the suicidal intent or motivation underlying the act. According to its latest annual report, 127 individuals under 18 years of age presented to hospital with self-harm, leading to 267 episodes of self-harm presentations in hospital (78). An even more striking gender difference was noted compared to that from the CDC, with 82.7% of the 127 individuals who presented to hospital in Oxford in 2012 being female.

2.5   Natural History and Outcome of Self-Harm

Despite the limited research investigating self-harm in early teens, self-harm onset is traditionally estimated to typically occur in this age group around the age of 14 years old (79, 80). Not much is known about the natural history and long-term outcomes of self-harm in adolescents, as longitudinal studies in this area remain relatively rare. A notable exception of this is a 25-year longitudinal study of a birth cohort consisting of 1,265 New Zealand children (81). After adjusting for confounding factors, it found that suicide attempts in adolescence were significantly associated with increased risks of subsequent suicide attempts (OR = 17.8), subsequent suicidal ideation (OR = 5.7) and major depression (OR = 1.5) in later life. Suicidal ideation without suicide attempt was significantly associated with slightly smaller increases in each of the three aforementioned outcomes as well. In females, suicidal behaviour in adolescence also increased risks of substance misuse in later life.

These findings where self-harm in adolescence is associated with negative mental health-related outcomes in later life are supported by a recent UK study based on Avon Longitudinal Study of Parents and Children (ALSPAC) birth cohort of children born in 1991 – 1992 (82). It involved 4,799 adolescents aged about 16 and found that self-harm at that age with or without suicidal intent was associated with an increased risk of self-harm, mental health problems and substance misuse in early adulthood. The increased risks were more strongly associated with suicidal versus non-suicidal self-harm. Suicidal self-harm only was also associated with poorer educational attainment and employment outcomes at age 19 years.

Evidence indicates that self-harm in adolescence is associated with elevated risks of subsequent self-harm episodes and suicide. For example, from a 20-year cohort study of 5,459 hospital patients who presented with self-harm at the age of 15 – 24 during 1978 – 1997, approximately a quarter

(26.3%) had a previous history of deliberate self-harm and 2.9% died during the follow-up period up till the end of 2000 (83). Of those who died, over half (57.4%) were probable suicides, representing a suicide risk approximately 10 times higher than expected based on national data for the age group. This contrasts somewhat with a longitudinal study examining the intra-individual suicide risk for individuals in 1994, 1997 and 2001 at the mean ages of 13, 16 and 20 years old respectively (84). In this study the intra-individual suicide risk was surprisingly stable during the adolescent years.

It appears that self-harm in adolescents decreases in frequency in late adolescence and may resolving spontaneously over time, as suggested by one unique population-based study that examined self-harming behaviour during the transition period between late adolescence and adulthood (85). As part of this study, a cohort of adolescents aged 14 – 15 years at recruitment participated in 9 chronological waves of data collection, which were conducted from years 1992 – 2008. The first 6 waves formed the adolescent phase in 1992 – 1995 and the last 3 waves represented the young adult phase in 1998 – 2008. The prevalence of self-harm in the adolescent phase decreased consistently from 5.1% in wave 3 (mean age = 15.9 years) to 1.5% in wave 6 (mean age = 17.4 years). This trend continued into the young adult phase, with the prevalence of self-harm in wave 7 being 1.7% (mean age = 20.7 years), declining to 0.5% in wave 9 (mean age = 29.0 years).

2.6   Is Self-Harm Prevalence in Adolescents Increasing?

Self-harm prevalence in adolescents appears to have increased over the years, although the data is somewhat conflicting, largely due to the variations in methodology used and the characteristics of the adolescent sample population studied. It may be that the prevalence of attempted suicide has not changed substantially in contrast to the prevalence of self-harm overall.

Based on national youth surveys conducted every two years in the United States as part of the Youth Risk Behaviour Surveillance System (86), significant linear decreases in the prevalence of three out of the five suicide-related behaviours assessed by YRBSS was observed from 1991 – 2013 (87). The suicide-related behaviours were assessed for the 12 months prior to each survey in nationwide adolescent students in Grades 9 – 12. The three behaviours that appeared to decrease in prevalence over the years were having serious considerations for attempting suicide (from 29.0% to 17.0%), making a plan for suicide (from 18.6% to 13.6%), and attempting suicide itself (from 7.3% to 8.0%). Note that by comparing the proportion of students who attempted suicide in 1991 to that in 2013, there is a slight increase of 0.7% in attempted suicides. However, simply comparing the earliest and latest data points may not necessarily reflect the long-term trend during that time period. The researchers conducted logistic regression analyses that adjusted for sex, grade and ethnicity over time, and found an overall linear decrease in attempted suicides from 1991 to 2013. The other two suicide-related behaviours that showed no significant linear or quadratic trend during 1991 – 2013 and 1999 – 2013 were feeling sad or hopeless and having attempting suicide resulting in medical treatment by a doctor or nurse respectively. Neither of these behaviours had significant changes in prevalence between 2011 and 2013.

In spite of the decreasing linear trends in three of the five YRBSS-assessed suicide-related behaviours, quadratic trends have shown that the prevalence of those who seriously considered attempting suicide actually increased during 2009 – 2013 (13.8% – 17.0%), levelling off recently with no significant change in prevalence between 2011 (15.8%) and 2013 (17.0%). A similar trend was observed for the prevalence of those who made a suicide plan, increasing during 2009 – 2013 (10.9% – 13.6%), with no significant change between 2011 (12.8%) and 2013 (13.6%). The prevalence of attempted suicides did not show a similar quadratic trend over the years although it stabilised recently from 2011 (7.8%) to 2013 (8.0%).

On the other hand, focusing on NSSI, the latest review of self-harm prevalence in adolescent populations worldwide analysed data from published studies during 2005 – 2011 (35). The mean lifetime prevalence rate of NSSI in adolescents was shown to have increased from just below 10% in 2005 to being just below 20% in 2011. The mean lifetime prevalence rates of NSSI and DSH have remained relatively stable within the latter four years. Studies where repeat surveys were conducted over time in the same adolescent population to assess self-harm prevalence in general found a rise in self-harm prevalence in adolescents over time (88 – 91).

2.7   Completed Suicides in Adolescents

The link between self-harm and an elevated suicide risk in the future has been well established. According to a 25-year database of suicide in children and adolescents in Northern Finland (92), a significant proportion of suicide victims had a history of self-cutting (33% of females and 7% of males) and previous suicide attempts (25% of females and 4% of males). It is also estimated that the majority of children and adolescents who die of suicide meet diagnostic criteria for a psychiatric disorder and 30% have depressive symptoms at the time of death (93, 94).

According the World Health Organisation (WHO), it is estimated that there were 804,000 suicides worldwide in 2012, with suicide being the second leading cause of death in young people age 15 – 29 years old globally (95). Generally, suicide rates are lowest for the age group below 15 years old across almost every region of the world. There are consistent regional variations in suicide rates with Eastern European and Far Eastern countries having the highest rates (96). Evidence suggests that suicide methods are highly dependent on their availability and the victim's access to the method (97). For example a Korean study has found that the suicide rate in rural areas was higher than in urban areas but in urban areas, the rate of suicide by jumping from heights was significantly higher than that in rural areas due to the greatly increased availability and access to tall buildings (98). For children and adolescents, the most common methods of suicide are hanging, jumping from heights and railway-related suicides (99).

2.8   Summary

With the varied methodology and definitions of self-harm used in prevalence studies, establishing the true prevalence of self-harm in adolescents is full of challenges. The general consensus is that self-harm is common in young people (15 – 46% adolescents in the community according the latest international review), probably rising and associated with a range of negative psychological outcomes in adulthood. Whilst self-harm in adolescents tends to reduce significantly over time (85), a significant proportion of adolescents will continue to self-harm and some may eventually die of suicide.

3

The Genetics of Self-Harm

Genetic factors can influence the risk of engaging in self-harm, particularly with regards to suicidal self-harm. Suicidal behaviours often "run in families", which may be due to environmental factors as well as genetic factors. Much of the research in genetics and self-harm to date has focused on the phenotype of suicidal behaviours. Research into the genetics of NSSI remains in its infancy (100).

3.1   Familial Transmission of Suicidal Behaviour

In the quest to determine to what extent genetics and environment contribute to the aetiology of self-harm, three different types of study designs have been used, namely family studies, twin studies and adoption studies. They differ in their individual strengths and limitations.

Firstly, family studies are designed to assess the extent to which a given condition is transmitted within families (101). This is done by studying the extent to which the condition is expressed in different relatives of the affected individual ("proband"), as different relatives will vary in how close they are genetically and environmentally to the proband. The strengths of this type of study include that it can demonstrate familial clustering (i.e. when a significantly higher number of individuals within a family are affected relative to control individuals), characterise the extent and pattern of transmission, locating the origin of a disease in the family and hint at precursors to the development of a condition of interest. Its major limitation is that it cannot distinguish between the roles environmental factors and genetic factors play in the familial transmission pattern observed.

Family studies have helped to conclusively demonstrate that suicidal behaviour does cluster in and is transmitted within families (101). For example, the rate of suicide attempts in first-degree relatives of an adolescent suicide victim (suicide proband) has been shown to be higher relative to controls even after adjusting for familial psychiatric disorders (102). This is supported by a large population-based case control study, which found that suicide attempts by siblings (OR = 3.4) and parents (OR = 2.7 for mother, 1.9 for father) represent strong independent familial risk factors for youth suicide attempts (103). In that study, 20% of suicide attempts were linked to either familial psychopathology (13%) or familial suicide attempt (7%). A separate study examined the offspring of suicide attempters with and without siblings who also attempted suicide, noting that the there was a higher risk and earlier onset of suicide attempts in the offspring of suicide attempters with siblings concordant for suicide attempts relative to those without such siblings (104). More recently, a systematic review and meta-analysis determined that this familial aggregation of suicidal behaviour extends from suicide attempts to suicide completions as well (105). It determined that offspring of parents who died of suicide were almost twice as likely to die of suicide themselves relative to control offspring of two living parents (OR after adjusting for confounders = 1.94, 95% CI = 1.54 – 2.45). A similarly increased risk for suicide attempts was noted for children of parents who attempted suicide (OR after adjusting for confounders = 1.95, 95% CI = 1.48 – 2.57).

Twin studies are studies where participants consist of monozygotic or dizygotic twin pairs. The former type of twin pair share nearly 100% of their genes, whereas the latter type shares only about 50% of their genes. By comparing not only the twins within each pair, but also comparing the concordance of phenotypes between the two types of twin pairs, this allows for the investigation of and the differentiation between shared genetic and environmental factors that may contribute to a particular phenotype of interest.

A meta-analysis and systematic review of twin studies investigating the genetics of suicide found that the concordance for completed suicide was much higher in monozygotic twin pairs versus dizygotic twin pairs (106). The review estimated that based on epidemiological studies, the heritability of suicidality (including ideation, plans and attempts) is in the range of 30 – 55% and that the heritability is largely independent of that of psychiatric disorders. Although Voracek and Loibl (106) acknowledged that personal experiences of each twin not shared with the other twin do contribute significantly to the risk of suicidality, it is likely that a genetic predisposition to an increased risk of suicidality exists. The rate of suicide attempts in suicide survivors whose twin died of suicide is much higher in monozygotic versus dizygotic twins, whereas the rate of suicide attempts in non-suicide twin survivors were similar between monozygotic and dizygotic twin pairs (107). There was no difference in suicidal ideation prevalence between the bereaved mono- and dizygotic twins, although twins who were particularly close to their deceased co-twin (whether monozygotic or dizygotic) were more likely to have suicidal ideation. Given that the closeness of the twin relationship was unrelated to the rate of suicide attempts, this suggests that the genetic predisposition to suicidality applies only to suicide attempts and not suicidal ideation. This notion is supported by a separate community-based study that found maternal suicide attempt (but not maternal suicidal ideation) was associated with a significantly higher risk of suicide attempt in the offspring and at an earlier age (108).

A recent study of classical twin design found common genetic factors that underpinned NSSI and suicidal ideation, suggesting that the two phenomena may share similarities in their biological aetiology (109). Using a bivariate genetic model, genetic factors were found to account for a large part of the variance in NSSI (37% in men and 59% in women) and suicidal ideation (41% in men and 55% in women). A positive correlation between the two variables was also noted (r = 0.49 in men and r = 0.61 in women). However, this study is one of the few to investigate the genetics of NSSI and this territory remains largely unexplored.

Twin studies are not without limitations. They assume that twins (monozygotic or dizygotic) raised in the same homes will share identical or very similar environments, which is not always the case. In addition, the premise and main strength of twin studies lie in differentiating between genes and environment, thus inherently disregarding gene-environment interactions (110).

Similar to twin studies, adoption studies are another type of study used to investigate genetic and environmental factors that may influence a condition of interest. They are less commonly used than the two aforementioned study designs, possibly due to the increasing emphasis placed on privacy laws and in particular, on protecting the privacy of the biological parents. Adoption studies involve comparing the proband (usually the adoptee) with other control adoptees and the biological relatives of the proband. Adoption and suicide attempts have been linked (7.3% in adoptees vs. 3.1% in non-adoptees), even after adjusting for family income, parental education and the impulsivity of the adolescent adoptee (111). However, this was contradicted by a comprehensive review done in 2007 on adoption studies in this area (112). The review only included 3 existing adoption studies that looked at suicide. It concluded that suicide does indeed run in biological families when looking at adoptees who killed themselves (RR = 8.38, p = 0.0002), but not in the demographically matched, still-alive, healthy control adoptees. This suggests that there is most likely a strong genetic component in suicidal behaviour, which is independent of whether the individual is adopted or not. This was supported by more recent evidence, where data from the Danish Adoption Registry showed a significantly increased risk of suicide attempts in full siblings of adoptees who attempted suicides before the age of 60, relative to full siblings of adoptees who never attempted suicide (113). This finding remained significant after adjusting for the psychiatric history of the siblings (incidence rate ratio = 3.88, 95% CI = 1.42 – 10.6).

A closely related study using data from the Danish Adoption Registry reported similar findings for the risk of suicide – with a significantly increased risk of suicide in full siblings of adoptees who died of suicide before the age of 60 versus full siblings of adoptees who did not die of suicide (114). Again, this was independent of psychiatric disorders (incidence rate ratio = 4.19, 95% CI = 1.00 – 17.5). Like that of suicide attempts, the increased risk of suicide has been shown to be independent of whether the proband was adopted or not. In a large Swedish national cohort study, the hazard ratios for suicide in the offspring of parents who died of suicide were similar comparing adopted offspring and non-adopted offspring even after adjusting for sex, age and socioeconomic factors (115).

3.2   Molecular Genetics of Suicidal Behaviour

With advances in molecular biology and genetics, studying and identifying genes at a molecular level has become increasingly possible. One popular and powerful tool used to investigate relations between conditions and genes is in the form of candidate-gene association studies; also known as CGAS (116). CGAS focus on investigating the associations between genetic variation within specific pre-selected genes ("candidate" genes) and certain phenotypes of interest (in this case, suicidal behaviour as a phenotype). Candidate genes from a range of neurobiological systems (e.g. serotonergic system, dopaminergic system, etc.) have been studied.

Given the complexity of the phenotype of suicidal behaviour, it may be much easier and more practical to link genotype with intermediate phenotypes (117), such as impulsivity and pathological aggression, and make inferences from there of the pathway between genotype and suicidal behaviour. This concept of intermediate phenotypes or "endophenotypes" can be defined as "measurable components unseen by the unaided eye along the pathway between disease and distal genotype" (118). Research into endophenotypes and suicidal behaviour remains in its infancy, but some of the most promising endophenotypes of suicidal behaviour to date are impulsivity, aggression and early-onset major depression (119). In particular, impulsivity has been linked to repeated episodes of self-harm (120).

3.3   The Serotonergic System

The serotonergic system plays an important role in impulse control (121, 122), as well as mood (123), both of which are key aspects of suicidal behaviour. The system has therefore been investigated the most thoroughly out of all the neurotransmitter systems that have been studied in relation to suicidal behaviour. Significant abnormalities in the serotonergic system, including variations from the tryptophan hydroxylase gene to the serotonin transporter (5-HTT) gene, have been found to be associated with suicidal behaviour (124). An overview of the conclusions from the latest systematic review of serotonergic genes and suicidal behaviour (125) is presented in Table 3.1.

The associations between tryptophan hydroxylase (TPH1 &TPH2 gene polymorphisms) and suicidal behaviour have been confirmed by further studies (126 – 128). In addition, a systematic review and meta-analysis focusing on genetic polymorphisms (specifically serotonin transporter polymorphisms) and suicide attempts in patients with mental disorders was published (129). An association between serotonin-transporter-linked polymorphisms and suicide was determined, with the relationship being strongest for those with bipolar disorder, major depression and schizophrenia (129).

Gene	Normal Function of Gene Product	Relation to Suicidal Behaviour
Serotonin Transporter (5-HTT)	Uptake of serotonin from synaptic cleft	5-HTTLPR polymorphism associated with violent suicidal behaviour relatively consistently in Caucasian populations (less consistent in non-Caucasians)
Serotonin Receptors (HTR1A, HTR2A)	Serotonin neurotransmission	No consistent association. Mostly negative associations for HTR1A. Inconsistent results for HTR2A variants
Tryptophan Hydroxylase (TPH1 & TPH2)	Rate-limiting enzyme responsible for serotonin synthesis	Link between TPH1 and suicidality - A218C/A779C polymorphisms linked to suicide in Caucasians. No consistent association between THP2 alleles and attempted/completed suicide
Monoamine Oxidase A (MAOA)	Mitochondrial enzyme responsible for serotonin degradation	No evidence indicating direct link between MAOA and suicidality. MAOA variation (e.g. in promoter region) linked to impulsivity and aggression
Gene-environment Interactions		5-HTTLPR, MAOA and HTR2A variants shown to interact with stressful life events, increasing risk of engaging in suicidal behaviour

Table 3.1: Serotonergic Genes and Suicidal Behaviour.

3.4   The Noradrenergic and Dopaminergic Systems

Unlike serotonin, far fewer studies are available on the possible implications of either the noradrenergic or the dopaminergic systems in suicidal behaviour, although abnormalities in both the noradrenergic and the dopaminergic systems have been linked to self-harm (130).

According to one of the few reviews done on the noradrenergic system and suicidal behaviour (131), two areas that post-mortem studies have focused on are the tyrosine hydroxylase (TH) and noradrenergic receptor (particularly alpha-2A-adrenergic receptors) genes. TH is the rate-limiting enzyme of catecholamine synthesis (132). Since both noradrenaline and dopamine are catecholamines, tyrosine hydroxylase plays a key role in the synthesis of both neurotransmitters. The review of post-mortem studies concluded that TH expression and alpha-2A-adrenergic receptor expression are both typically increased in the brains of suicide victims relative to normal controls (131). TH gene variants (rs3842727, rs6356) have been studied but no clear associations between them and suicide or suicide-related traits have been found in a relatively large study of 571 suicide attempters and normal controls (133).

Single nucleotide polymorphisms (SNPs) of the alpha-2A-adrenergic receptor gene have garnered attention for possible associations with suicidal behaviour. Three such SNPs (C-1291G, N251K, rs3750625C/A) were investigated in a sample of 184 Japanese suicide victims relative to control subjects (134). The study found mixed results, with the N251K SNP having no significant association with suicide at all but the C-1291G SNP having a significant association with suicide for females only (p=0.043 and 0.013 for genotypic and allelic comparisons respectively). For male suicides, whether violent or otherwise, neither of these 2 SNPs demonstrated any association with suicide.

Studies have also looked at the genes related to DOPA decarboxylase (r1451371, rs1470750, rs99885), the enzyme responsible for a range of decarboxylation reactions including the conversion of L-DOPA (precursor of dopamine, noradrenaline and adrenaline) to dopamine. There were marginal associations found between DOPA decarboxylase variants (r1451371, rs1470750) and non-violent suicide attempts, but this was coupled with several negative findings – DOPA decarboxylase genotypes or haplotypes were not associated with suicidal behaviour and DOPA decarboxylase SNPs were not associated with impulsive suicide attempts (133). This study overall offers weak evidence for possible associations between DOPA decarboxylase variants and violent suicidal behaviour.

Whilst DOPA decarboxylase may only be weakly associated with suicidal behaviour, a more substantial body of evidence exists for another enzyme called catechol-O-methyltransferase (COMT), which is responsible for the inactivation of both dopamine and noradrenaline. Most studies in the area have focused on one particular functional polymorphism in the COMT gene called Val158Met, which is easily detectable and has been implicated in the pathogenesis of a range of mental disorders including schizophrenia, bipolar disorder and obsessive-compulsive disorder (135). A meta-analysis (136) collated data from 6 studies and noted a significant association between the COMT Val158Met polymorphism and suicidal behaviour (OR = 1.25, 95% CI = 1.01 – 1.56, p=0.04). Although no publication bias was detected, careful analysis of the data collated for this meta-analysis showed that the positive association was highly dependent on the inclusion of all of the studies, because when 5 of the 6 studies were removed individually and systematically from the analysis, the association was no longer significant. Careful interpretation of this meta-analysis is needed as this suggests that the relationship observed between COMT and suicidal behaviour was not robust. The latest meta-analysis, which specifically focused on COMT genes and suicidal behaviour (137) concluded that there was no direct association between COMT variants and suicidal behaviour. The conclusion of this meta-analysis is in line with a previous meta-analysis that looked at the COMT polymorphism Val158Met specifically (138).

Despite the lack of a direct association between COMT variants and suicidal behaviour, certain COMT variants have been associated with particular personality traits that may be key endophenotypes worth investigating further. The COMT Val/Val genotype has been significantly associated with impulsive behaviour and psychiatric disorders in suicide attempters (139). It has also been associated with anger-related traits. In one study of suicide attempters, the Val/Val genotype was more commonly found in the suicide attempter group versus that in the normal control group (140). In addition, the Val/Val genotype was associated with higher scores for anger traits as measured by the State-Trait Anger Expression Inventory (STAXI) but only in female suicide attempters, indicating a possible gender difference in the association between Val/Val genotypes and anger. Some evidence suggests that this potential gender difference may apply to associations between COMT polymorphisms and traits beyond anger, such as anxiety (141). A study of patients with alcohol dependence whom attempted suicide noted that a higher frequency of the Met allele (as opposed to the Val allele from the aforementioned study) was found in male suicide attempters, with higher aggression and depression scores relative to male non-attempters (142). This suggests that COMT alleles may have different effects on individuals depending on gender. COMT variants remain a worthwhile area for further research to determine any associations they may have with endophenotypes related to suicidal behaviour.

Finally, an additional element of the dopaminergic system has been investigated for possible associations with suicidal behaviour. Two studies investigated the dopamine receptor subtype 4 (DRD4) gene exon III 48 bp repeat polymorphism. Though neither study found any associations between the DRD4 polymorphism and suicidal behaviour (143, 144), one of the studies noted that there was a significant difference in depression severity between adolescent suicidal inpatients who were homozygotes versus those who were heterozygotes for the DRD4 alleles (144). This latter observation suggests that like COMT polymorphisms, DRD4 polymorphisms may not be linked directly to suicidal behaviour, but instead to endophenotypes such as depression, novelty seeking and impulsivity (145).

This notion is supported by a recent review, which noted that certain genetic variants (including the serotonin transporter 5-HTTLPR polymorphism, COMT Val158Met and a variant of the dopamine receptor D2) may contribute to emotion dysregulation in children and adolescents (146). Although findings from individual studies have been inconsistent, it is plausible that emotion dysregulation could be an intermediate phenotype for suicidal behaviour, increasing one's susceptibility to suicidal behaviour.

3.5   Neurotrophic Factors

Neurotrophins or neurotrophic factors can be defined as a collection of "closely related proteins that were first identified as survival factors for sympathetic and sensory neurons", that are involved in the survival, development and function of neurons in both the central and peripheral nervous systems (147). One particular neurotrophin that has attracted attention in relation to suicidal behaviour is the brain-derived neutrophic factor (BDNF), the most abundant and widely present neurotrophic factor in the brain (148). A down-regulation of BDNF expression and BDNF's receptor tyrosine kinase B (TrkB) in the pre-frontal cortex and hippocampus has been observed in adolescent suicide victims versus normal control subjects (149). Similar findings have been replicated in other studies (150), and persist even when adjusted for psychiatric diagnoses, post-mortem interval, age, sex and the pH of the brain (151).

The mechanisms behind this down-regulation of BDNF expression are unclear. Recently, a hypothesis that an increase in DNA methylation in the BDNF promoter region could lead to the dysregulation of BDNF gene expression often observed in the brains of suicide victims has emerged. In a post-mortem study of the Wernicke's area in the brains of 44 White suicide victims compared to 33 White non-suicide control subjects, hyper-methylation of the BDNF promoter region was observed more frequently in suicide subjects compared to controls, independent of the genome-wide methylation levels (152). A subsequent smaller study led by the same researcher confirmed the hyper-methylation of the BDNF promoter region in the Wernicke's area in the brains of suicide subjects versus controls and also noted a lack of correlation between TrkB gene methylation in Wernicke's area and suicidal behavior (153). As well as being associated with completed suicides, hyper-methylation of the BDNF promoter region has been associated with a history of suicide attempts and suicidal ideation in patients with depression even when receiving antidepressant treatment (154). Similar correlations with suicidal ideation have been replicated in other studies (155, 156).

Of the BDNF gene, studies have focused on one particular SNP called Val66Met, which has been linked to anxiety (157), neuroticism (158) and depression (159). This Val/Met polymorphism of the BDNF gene has been associated with suicidal behaviour. Studies have found this association in bipolar patients (160) and in depressed patients (161). It has been shown in depressed patients to be an independent risk factor for high lethality in suicide attempts (162). However, a relatively large study of 512 suicide cases contradicts these findings, because it found that there was no significant association between the BDNF Val66Met polymorphism and completed suicide (163). It may be that the associations between BDNF Val66Met and suicide differ, depending on whether it is suicide attempts or completed suicides being investigated.

The Met allele in particular has been associated with several factors that may increase an individual's risk of engaging in suicidal behaviour. These factors include cognitive function (164), rumination (165), as well as the use of avoidant coping strategies after adjusting for age and depression

(166). A recent meta-analysis showed that the Met allele of the SNP was associated with an increased risk of suicide and a history of suicide attempts (167). A large study of 359 suicide victims compared with 201 control subjects found that the BDNF Val66Met SNP was associated with violent suicide for females and with suicide for those exposed to childhood trauma (168). The latter association with subjects who have experienced childhood maltreatment complements the findings from previous studies, including one that found an association between childhood trauma and violent suicide attempts in adults with the Val/Val genotype (169). Another found an association between the Met/Met and Met/Val genotypes of the Val66Met polymorphism and violent suicide in females, as well as in individuals who were exposed to childhood trauma (170).

Overall, it is not entirely clear how BDNF relates to the aetiology of adolescent suicidal behaviour but BDNF signalling abnormalities (151) and dysregulation (171) are likely to be involved. Whilst most studies have focused on suicidality and not NSSI, a rare and unique retrospective study investigated the BDNF genotype and self-injurious behaviour with or without suicidal intent (172). It found an association between childhood emotional environments as measured using the Childhood Trauma Questionnaire and self-harm behaviour for homozygous Val/Val individuals only and not for Met allele carriers. For those who had poor, invalidating childhood emotional environments, individuals with the homozygous Val/Val genotype were more likely than Met carriers to have a history of self-injurious behaviour with suicidal intent. On the other hand, for those who had supportive childhood emotional environments, Met carriers were more likely than homozygous Val/Val individuals to have a history of self-injurious behaviour, regardless of the presence or absence of suicidal intent. These findings support the theory that epigenetic changes and gene-environment interactions are important elements in the pathophysiology of suicidal behaviour. The association between hyper-methylation of the BDNF gene and suicidal behaviour also supports this theory (173, 174). Nevertheless, future research is needed to characterise the role of BDNF genes and BDNF-related epigenetic changes play in the pathophysiology of suicidal behaviour.

3.6   Summary

In summary, evidence gathered from adoption, twin and family studies point towards genetics being a key factor in the aetiology of suicidal behaviour. There is a distinct lack of such studies relating to non-suicidal self-injury, so future research is warranted to investigate if and how genetic factors play a role in the aetiology of non-suicidal self-injury as well. Development in the field of molecular genetics has allowed a number of candidate genes to be identified and studied in relation to suicidal behaviour. Of the candidate genes, the most consistent evidence has emerged from those related to the serotonergic system, although studies with larger sample sizes are still needed to confirm the initial findings. Evidence of the role of other candidate genes related to the noradrenergic and dopaminergic system in the aetiology of suicidal behaviour is lacking and far less consistent when compared to that available for the serotonergic system. Developing more refined definitions for the phenotype of self-harm behaviour may help identify small gene effects and help differentiate findings related to suicidal and non-suicidal self-harm, as currently the majority of the studies do not differentiate between the two. Future work should build on the studies that investigated candidate genes and their relationships to endophenotypes of self-harm.

4

Neurobiology and Self-Harm

Our understanding of the neurobiology of self-harm and suicidal behaviour in particular, has improved greatly over the past 30 years. Most of the research in this field has focused largely on suicidal behaviour in adults, although in recent years, there has been increasing interest in the neurobiology of NSSI and adolescent suicide. The methodology used in the field often relies on the post-mortem examination of brains of suicide victims though more recently, the use of neuroimaging techniques such as functional magnetic resonance imaging (fMRI) has been increasingly popular. Some of the neurobiological findings related to self-harm, such as an increased binding of the serotonin receptor 5-HT2A in the brain in suicide victims versus control subjects (175), can also be linked to our understanding of the genetics of suicidal behaviour, which is discussed in the previous chapter.

4.1   The Serotonergic System

Serotonin, also known as 5-hydroxytryptamine (5-HT), is an important monoamine neurotransmitter known for numerous functions including the regulation of mood. It has been implicated in relation to suicidal behaviour. A relatively consistent finding over the years has been an association between low levels of 5-hydroxyindoleacetic acid (5-HIAA), a major serotonin metabolite, in cerebrospinal fluid (CSF) and suicidal behaviour (176). This finding has been noted across cohorts with varying psychiatric diagnoses from schizophrenia (177) to mood disorders (178), suggesting that this finding is independent of psychiatric disorders. CSF 5-HIAA levels have been found to be typically lower in suicide attempters versus healthy controls (179), even after adjusting for age, co-morbid depression and substance abuse (180). Evidence suggests that CSF 5-HIAA levels may be a better predictor of suicide risk in males who have previously attempted suicide than the standard Beck Suicide Intent Scale or the Beck Hopelessness Scale (181). Low CSF 5-HIAA concentrations have also been associated with violent, aggressive behaviour and loss of impulse control in primate models (182). This has been replicated in human studies as well, where CSF 5-HIAA levels have been shown to be lower in impulsive than in non-impulsive violent suicide attempters (183). This link to impulsivity and aggression or violence may be part of the mechanism behind which low CSF 5-HIAA levels possibly increase an individual's susceptibility and risk of engaging in suicidal behaviour.

Serotonin receptor dysfunction has been shown to be linked to suicidal behaviour. The focus of research in this field has largely been on 5-HT2A receptors. A greater expression of serotonin receptor 2A (5-HT2A) in the prefrontal cortex and hippocampus, brain regions that are linked to cognition and stress, have been found in post-mortem teenage suicide victims' brains relative to matched controls (184). This finding has been noted to be one of the most consistent post-mortem biological abnormalities found in suicide victims (185). It may be linked to a significantly lower binding potential of the pre-frontal 5-HT2A receptors, which has been noted in patients who have attempted suicide versus normal controls (186). There is also a positive correlation between lifetime aggression scores and pre-frontal 5-HT2A receptor binding in post-mortem studies of suicide victims, which does not exist in the brains of non-suicide subjects (187). Even after adjusting for age, this decrease in serotonin 5-HT2A receptor binding capability persists remains in vivo (188). It is more prominent in self-injury patients versus self- poisoning patients (188).

In addition to studies investigating 5-HT2A receptors in the brain, other studies have investigated 5-HT2A receptors in platelets. This is viewed as one of a range of peripheral serotonergic markers in the body. It has been hypothesised that platelet 5-HT2A receptor binding and tryptophan availability may be linked in some way to suicidality. One large study, however, has found no significant differences in 5-HT2A receptor binding in platelets or plasma tryptophan/amino acids between those who have had a recent suicide attempt and controls with no previous suicide attempt (189). This was followed by another study, which looked at 5 different peripheral serotonergic markers (platelet serotonin concentration, serotonin uptake activity, 5-HT2A receptor binding characteristics, MAO-B activity and plasma tryptophan concentration) in suicide attempters, non-suicidal patients with major depression, and healthy control volunteers (190). Mean platelet serotonin concentrations for non-suicidal depressed subjects were much higher than that for suicide attempters and healthy controls, which were the same. Mean K_D (dissociation constant) for the platelet 5-HT2A receptor and MAO-B activity was significantly lower in suicidal subjects relative to control; however this may have been linked to depression rather than suicidal behaviour as the difference was no longer significant when comparing suicidal subjects with non-suicidal depressed patients. Mean V_{max} of serotonin uptake (in washed platelets only, not in platelet-rich plasma) was significantly higher in suicidal patients versus healthy controls, a difference that similarly disappears when comparing suicidal subjects with non-suicidal depressed patients. Gender differences within the group of suicide attempters were also observed for some of the peripheral markers – for female suicide attempters, they had lower MAO-B activity and for male suicide attempters, they had higher V_{max} of serotonin uptake in washed platelets. Whilst such studies on peripheral serotonergic markers do provide valuable information, the actual significance of them in relation to the function of the central nervous system (CNS) is not very clear at the moment (191). More research is needed in the future to clarify this somewhat confusing collection of evidence to date.

One other element of the serotonergic system that has been investigated in relation to suicidal behaviour is the serotonin transporter (5-HTT) in the brain, responsible for serotonin re-uptake at synaptic clefts which therefore influences serotonin neurotransmission. Most of the studies done have used post-mortem examination of brains of suicide victims, and have focused most commonly on the front cortex region of the brain. The role of 5-HTT in the pathophysiology of suicide has remained unclear since the publication of a review on this topic in 2003 (192). It has been found that there is a diffuse reduction in 5-HTT binding in the pre-frontal cortex (PFC) of patients with major depression (193). In the same post-mortem study, a localised reduction in 5-HTT binding was also found specifically in the ventral PFC of suicide victims relative to non-suicide controls and subjects with major depression (193). Since the publication of that study, neuroimaging studies have identified reductions in 5-HTT binding in specific regions of the brain, which have been associated with various conditions including obsessive-compulsive disorder (194) and recreational ecstasy abuse (195). These studies collectively suggest that the level of 5-HTT binding in specific regions of the brain may be linked to certain mental disorders and possibly also to suicidal behaviour, but more research is needed in the future to clarify and confirm this.

According to the latest review on serotonin and suicidal behaviour (196), results from adult and adolescent studies have been mixed and conflicting. A recent review on NSSI noted similarly conflicting evidence for associations between serotonin and NSSI, although it stated that some evidence existed for an association between serotonin deficiency and self-harm (197). The latter review pointed out one study that found the level of peripheral serotonin, conflict in the mother-child relationship and interactions with negativity to account for up to 64% of the variance in self-injury in adolescents (198), suggesting that serotonin does play a significant role in the neurobiological basis of self-harm. From the evidence base available, it is clear that serotonergic dysfunction is linked to self-harm, independent of psychiatric co-morbidities (199). The precise mechanisms and details behind the associations remain poorly understood to date.

4.2   The Hypothalamic-Pituitary-Adrenal (HPA) Axis

The hypothalamic-pituitary-adrenal (HPA) axis is a term used to describe the complex relationship and feedback system that exist between three endocrine glands, namely the hypothalamus, the pituitary gland and the adrenal glands. The HPA axis is a key part of the neuroendocrine system and plays a major role in regulating the body's response to stress. Normally, in response to stress, the hypothalamus would secrete corticotropin-releasing hormone (CRH), which upon binding at receptors on the anterior pituitary gland triggers the release of adrenocorticotropic hormone (ACTH) from the pituitary gland. ACTH then binds to its receptors on the adrenal cortex of the adrenal glands and stimulates the release of the hormone cortisol from the adrenal glands. The increase in cortisol eventually completes the negative feedback loop by inhibiting the release of CRH and ACTH from the hypothalamus and the pituitary gland respectively.

Due to the HPA axis' intimate relationship with the body's stress response, HPA dysfunction has been implicated in the neurobiology underlying a variety of mood disorders, including major depression (200) and bipolar disorder (201). Hypercortisolaemia, an abnormally elevated level of cortisol and a common feature of HPA axis dysfunction, has been linked to the pathophysiology of depressive symptoms and cognitive deficits often observed in severe mood disorders (202).

For suicidality, most of the data available regarding the HPA axis arises from studies that used the dexamethasone suppression test (DST) to assess the HPA negative feedback system (203). Dexamethasone is an exogenous steroid, of which a dose is injected into a subject as part of the DST. The dose of dexamethasone mimics an increase in endogenous glucocorticoid levels. Like endogenous glucocorticoids would, dexamethasone binds to glucocorticoid receptors on the anterior pituitary gland to suppress the secretion of ACTH, which then leads to a reduction in cortisol release from adrenal glands downstream. As a way of assessing adrenal function and the negative feedback system part of the HPA axis, subjects whose endogenous cortisol production is not suppressed in response to the DST are often referred to "non-suppressors" and their "DST-positive" result may indicate certain underlying pathologies.

A mixture of associations between HPA axis function, suicidal behaviour and suicidal ideation has been found across the few studies done in this area over the years. One of the earliest of such studies was one that examined the plasma cortisol response pre- and post-DST in 49 prepubertal psychiatric inpatient children to determine if there are any associations between HPA axis function, of which DST results were used as an index, and suicidality (204). In this study, modest associations were found between suicidality, ranging from suicidal ideation to suicide attempts, and plasma cortisol measurements, independent of psychiatric diagnosis. These associations were only found for pre-DST cortisol measurements and not that measured post-DST. Another study conducted DST in adolescents with major depressive disorder and found that there was no correlation between the cortisol response to DST and factors including suicidality, psychotic symptoms, inpatient status or a history of major depressive disorder (205).

One recent study investigated the HPA axis in relation to adolescents engaging in NSSI (206). It found a statistically significant difference in the cortisol response between those engaging in NSSI and healthy controls, with the NSSI group having a lower mean cortisol response than the control group. The results of this study tentatively suggest that hypofunction of the HPA axis is associated with NSSI behaviour in adolescents, with the reduced cortisol secretion possibly increasing adolescent vulnerability to maladaptive stress responses. This finding complements that from another study, which found that lower post-DST cortisol was independently associated with current suicidal ideation and past self-inflicted injury in female adolescents with a history of depression with or without self-harm (207). The results of this latter study appear to link post-DST cortisol suppression with suicide, contradicting previous reports of associations between post-DST cortisol non-suppression and suicide in adult samples (208 – 210).

Overall, a significant body of evidence exists supporting the notion of HPA axis hyperactivity being linked to suicidal behaviour (211 – 215) as well as some evidence (206, 207) suggesting that low HPA axis activity may be linked to suicidal behaviour (216), albeit the latter side being less compelling (217). In addition to the effects caused by HPA dysfunction itself, the HPA's complicated relationships with the noradrenergic and dopaminergic systems mean that HPA dysfunction will have an impact on both of these monoamine systems as well (202, 218).

4.3   The Noradrenergic System

There is limited evidence available regarding neurobiological abnormalities of the noradrenergic system relating to suicidal behaviour. One of the early key observations made was that there were fewer pigmented noradrenergic neurons in the post-mortem examination of the locus coeruleus of suicide victims versus controls with no psychiatric or neurologic disorder (219). Since the locus coeruleus (LC) is the primary source of noradrenaline in the brain and is involved with physiological responses to stress, it was hypothesised that chronic, long-term activation of LC due to chronic stress would lead to a depletion in synaptic noradrenaline, ultimately leading to compensatory changes in noradrenergic neurons in the LC of suicide victims (220). This hypothesis was supported by the post-mortem observation that there was an elevated expression of tyrosine hydroxylase (TH) in the LC in subjects with major depression, most of whom died by suicide (221). Since tyrosine hydroxylase is the rate-limiting enzyme in the synthesis of catecholamines including noradrenaline, this finding would suggest that those depressed subjects had hyper-activity of the noradrenergic neurons in the LC or a deficiency of noradrenaline itself in the LC.

Though these observations support the implication of noradrenergic dysfunction in the pathophysiology of suicidal behaviour, other studies contradict these observations. A post-mortem study used immunostaining and found no significant differences in the number of tyrosine hydroxylase neurons between depressed suicide victims and controls (222), suggesting that noradrenergic function of the LC does not differ greatly between suicide and non-suicide subjects. The same study noted that the number of tyrosine hydroxylase immuno-reactive neurons were associated negatively with the mean dose of antidepressants taken, suggesting that antidepressants may regulate the noradrenergic activity of the LC and that the noradrenergic observations made are related to depression instead of suicidal behaviour. The finding that the noradrenergic activity of the LC may be related to depression is in line with that of previous studies (223 – 225). Overall, findings related to tyrosine hydroxylase immune-cyto-chemical staining density have been conflicting in studies of suicide victims compared to matched control subjects (203).

On the other hand, lower levels of 3-methoxy-4-hydroxyphenyl-glycol (MHPG), an important noradrenaline metabolite, in cerebrospinal fluid (CSF) have been associated with self-rated depression severity and the short-term risk of future suicidal behaviour in the year of follow-up immediately after a major depressive episode, based on a study of 184 patients with major depressive or bipolar disorder (226). CSF monoamine metabolite levels including 5-HIAA, homovanillic acid (key metabolite of catecholamines including dopamine in the brain) and MHPG all showed a negative correlation with the lethality of suicide attempts during a 2-year follow-up study of patients with bipolar disorder (227). This suggests that CSF monoamine metabolite levels may offer clinically relevant predictions of the risk of engaging in future suicidal behaviour. This is supported by the findings of a recent study that investigated biological patterns among 20 different CSF biomarkers including homovanillic acid (HVA), 5-HIAA, chemokines, cytokines and MHPG, and their relations to suicidal behaviour in suicide attempters (228). The study found that a combination of monoamine metabolites (5-HIAA, HVA), the pro-inflammatory cytokine interleukin-6 (IL-6) and the HPA axis-related orexin in CSF were significantly associated with violent suicide attempts and the future risk of completed suicide.

4.4   The Dopaminergic System

Building on the aforementioned study that looked at 20 different biomarkers in CSF samples, a number of similar studies over the years have focused on the levels of homovanillic acid or HVA, a key metabolite of dopamine, in CSF as an index of dopaminergic activity, because they are directly influenced by dopamine metabolism in the brain. Yet this approach is not without limitations, as other factors outside of the dopaminergic system (e.g. rates of transport from CSF to blood, volume of ventricles where CSF is present, etc.) can affect the levels of HVA in CSF (229). The majority of studies have focused on suicidal behaviour, with only very limited evidence available linking the dopaminergic system to NSSI (197). One study that compared the levels of monoamine neurotransmitters including HVA in CSF samples from individuals with a history of repetitive NSSI found no significant difference in the levels observed when compared to diagnostically-matched individuals with no history of NSSI (230).

A significant body of evidence in the literature indicates that a lower CSF HVA concentration is often found in suicide attempters relative to control subjects with no history of suicide attempts. One study of 120 suicide attempters found that they had significantly lower HVA levels (174 ± 82 vs. 216 ± 96 nmol/L, p = 0.004), HVA: 5-HIAA and HVA: MHPG ratios than healthy controls (231). Similar results of significantly lower CSF HVA levels in suicide attempters versus controls with no history of suicide attempts has been shown in previous studies (232 – 234). However, one study of chronic schizophrenic patients did find that there was no significant difference in the mean CSF HVA concentration between suicide attempters (whether they were violent or non-violent suicide attempts) and controls with no history of suicide attempts (235). This study is isolated in its finding compared to other studies that have found a significant correlation.

HVA levels in CSF appeared to be associated with suicidal intent as measured by the Beck Suicide Intent Scale in suicide attempters (236). In a similar, subsequent study of suicide attempters, it was found that CSF HVA levels correlated with scores on the Beck Suicide Intent Scale only for non-violent suicide attempts ($r = -0.99$, $p < 0.024$) and not for violent suicides (237). CSF HVA levels showed no difference between high and low-lethality suicide attempters, and did not differentiate completed suicides and suicide survivors in the 5-year period. This complemented the findings of a separate study of 93 subjects presenting with a major depressive episode, where no significant associations between CSF HVA levels, aggression and suicidal behaviour were noted (238).

Tentatively, it would appear that CSF HVA levels tend to be lower in suicide attempters versus controls with no history of suicide attempts, but it is unclear whether this association extends to suicidal intent or the lethality of the act as well. Lower CSF HVA concentrations may suggest reduced dopamine levels and function in the brain, which has been associated with completed suicides (239) and suicide attempts but not the lethality of the act in depressed subjects (240). Similar findings regarding reduced dopaminergic function and suicide attempts have also been noted in non-depressed subjects (241). The clinical relevance of these findings remains unclear (203).

4.5   Endogenous Opioids and Pain Perception

In contrast to the majority of research done on the HPA axis, serotonergic, noradrenergic and dopaminergic systems that focused on suicidal self-harm, a significant proportion of research relating to the endogenous opioid system and pain perception has focused on NSSI.

The endogenous opioid system is a large and complex system that acts to provide an endogenous analgesic effect. There are 3 major classes of endogenous opioid peptides, namely β-endorphins, enkephalins and dynorphins, which act as neurotransmitters and neuromodulators by binding to opioid receptors (242). Opioid receptors can be split into three types, namely μ (mu), δ (delta) and κ (kappa) receptors. They are widely expressed in both the central and peripheral nervous system, and the peripheral opioid receptors in particular can be targeted for clinical pain management (243).

It has been shown in individuals who engage in NSSI that they tend to have significantly reduced CSF levels of β-endorphins and enkephalins, but similar levels of dynorphins when compared to individuals with no history of NSSI (230). Bresin & Gordon proposed a functional model of the pathophysiology of NSSI, where they hypothesised that individuals with a history of NSSI tend to have a lower resting level of β-endorphins and enkephalins with normal levels of dynorphins relative to individuals with no NSSI history (244). Coupled with this lower baseline level of endoge- nous opioids, the model proposes that NSSI behaviour itself triggers the release of endogenous opioids and the opioids released during NSSI regu- late affect, reducing negative affect that has been shown to lead to cravings for NSSI (245). Whilst a significant body of evidence has informed each part of the functional model proposed by Bresin & Gordon, they acknowledge that replication of the reviewed results they have collated is important and that their hypotheses remain to be validated (244).

Based on the evidence available, the relationship between the imbal- ance in the endogenous opioid system and NSSI remains a classic causality dilemma of "which came first", that is whether the NSSI behaviour caused the opioid imbalance observed or whether the opioid imbalance was pre- sent prior the start of NSSI behaviour and increased one's susceptibility to engaging in NSSI. To solve this dilemma, it is clear that longitudinal stud- ies are required in the future. Subject to future research, the endogenous opioid system may be a promising target for new therapeutic approaches in the treatment of NSSI patients. Some evidence has already indicated partial success of treating or at least ameliorating NSSI by the administra- tion of opioid antagonists (246).

Given that endogenous opioids play a key role in pain perception (247, 248), endogenous opioid imbalance is one possible explanation be- hind the altered pain perception often observed in individuals who engage in self-harm. Since the 1990s, evidence has emerged linking suicidal behav- iour and self-injurious behaviour with increased physical pain thresholds or endurance, as well as reduced pain sensitivity. Suicide attempters demonstrated a higher endurance to pain induced by electric shocks and reduced pain sensitivity relative to a control group of community individ- uals and relative to patients who presented to hospital with accidental in- juries (249). In this study, it was noted that the pain endurance of suicide attempters was associated with negative scores on psychological variables including stressful events, anxiety, depression, body image – the more negative the scores, the higher the pain endurance shown by the subject. A subsequent study found similar results, with suicidal inpatient adolescents demonstrating higher pain thresholds and tolerances to thermal pain stimuli compared to non-suicidal adolescent inpatients and healthy control participants (250). Some evidence suggests that the elevated pain threshold and tolerance seen in young adults who self-injure are associated with depression (251).

In addition to the reasonably consistent observations that individuals who engage in self-harm tend to have higher physical pain thresholds and endurance than individuals who do not engage in self-harm, there has been interest in how the altered pain perception relates to the emotional or psychological state of the individual. In a lab-based study using pressure on the finger as a pain stimulus, it was observed that participants with self-injury history had higher pain thresholds, with the longer the history, the higher the pain threshold (252). This study found that increased pain endurance was not related to self-injury history, but rather to elevated levels of introversion, neuroticism, negative beliefs about self-worth and a highly self-critical cognitive style. A self-critical cognitive style has also been implicated in a separate study of adolescent with self-injury as a mediator between NSSI, elevated pain thresholds and pain endurance (253). Building on this, elevated pain tolerance was observed in young adults with recent deliberate self-harm (DSH) when subjected to interpersonal distress, compared to that observed in controls without any history of DSH (254).

Together, these three studies support the hypothesis that emotion dysregulation is likely to play a key role in mediating the altered pain perception observed in individuals who engage in self-harm. This can be linked to evidence that indicate endogenous opioids modulate reward (255) and incentive motivational processes in the brain (256). This possible association between emotion dysregulation and altered pain perception has been demonstrated in a study of 72 young adults with and without NSSI (257). Whilst a positive correlation between emotion dysregulation as assessed by the Difficulties in Emotion Regulation Scale and diminished pain perception was indeed found, it was surprisingly found in both groups of participants, suggesting that the association between emotion dysregulation and altered pain perception may in fact be independent of self-harm behaviour.

Some studies have investigated the relationships between pain perception and self-harm behaviour in individuals with bipolar disorder (258, 259). Female bipolar patients who experience no pain during self-injury have been shown to have poorer discrimination of thermal stimuli of similar intensity compared to those who feel pain during self-injury and those with no history of self-harm (260). This 'analgesia' experienced by some bipolar patients is likely to be due to neurosensory changes and the pain response in female bipolar patients have been observed to be neurobiologically different from that in age-matched control subjects (261). In particular, there was a greater response in the dorsolateral pre-frontal cortex of the brain with a reduced response in the anterior cingulate and amygdala, generating a possible neurobiological mechanism behind the elevated pain thresholds observed in female bipolar individuals.

A study has shown that the altered pain perception seen with self-harm behaviour can normalise after the self-harm behaviour stops (262). This study was conducted in patients with borderline personality disorder. Those with current self-injurious behaviour demonstrated lower pain sensitivity than healthy controls and those with a history of such behaviour but no current self-harm.

In summary, abnormalities in the endogenous opioid system and pain perception have been of interest in individuals who engage in self-harm, and in particular NSSI. An imbalance in levels of endogenous opioids has been implicated in NSSI, although causality is yet to be established. The tenuous link for emotion dysregulation as a mediator of altered pain perception in individuals who engage in NSSI needs to be explored further, which could potentially validate the hypothesis that emotion regulation is one of the key functions of NSSI. There remains methodological challenges to be overcome in future research in the field. Studies investigating endogenous opioids and NSSI have been conducted entirely in clinical samples (244). Also, there have been no studies on endogenous opioids in self-injury ideation and limitations exist for the current methodology used to assess endogenous opioid activity (263). Advances in methodology must be made in order to truly test and validate the model of NSSI proposed by Bresin and Gordon. Future work must also extend to including community-based samples.

4.6   Signal Transduction Abnormalities

Abnormalities in signal transduction processes within cells have been proposed to be part of the aetiology of suicidal behaviour. Post-mortem examinations of the brains of suicide victims have proved to be a useful source of information in this area. Two particular enzymes have featured notably in studies: protein kinase A (PKA), an enzyme involved in the adenylyl cyclase signalling pathway, and protein kinase C (PKC), an enzyme involved in the phosphoinositide signalling system (264). Being protein kinase enzymes, both act to phosphorylate a range of transcription factors, influencing downstream gene expression.

One such transcription factor that has been linked to the pathophysiology of suicide is cyclic AMP response element binding protein (CREB). It is one of the main downstream target proteins of PKA (265). One study found significantly elevated levels of CREB in the brains of antidepressant drug-free depressed suicide subjects versus that in matched control subjects (266). This increase in CREB levels was not found in depressed suicide subjects who were treated with antidepressants. From this study, levels of PKA also correlated with levels of CREB in the pre-frontal cortex (PFC) of the depressed suicide subjects. This could be interpreted as a coordinated upregulation of cyclic AMP signalling demonstrated by the upregulation of both PKA and CREB in the PFC in depressed suicide victims. It is not very clear from the results of this study as to whether this upregulation is linked to depression or suicidal behaviour or both, but the fact that elevated CREB levels were only found in those depressed suicide victims who were free of antidepressant treatment suggests that cAMP signalling alterations are involved in the pathophysiology of depression instead of suicidal behaviour. Supporting the hypothesis that CREB may play an important role in the pathophysiology of depression, a study observed reduced CRE-DNA binding activity and CREB protein expression in the neutrophils of drug-free patients with major depressive disorder when compared to normal control subjects (267).

Other subsequent studies conducted have found contradictory results, with most of them noting a decrease in CREB and PKA levels in the brains of suicide victims. One such study included 17 suicide victims, observing a reduced number of [3H] cAMP binding sites for PKA and significantly reduced PKA activity in the presence and absence of cAMP in the

PFC of suicide victims, compared to that in non-psychiatric control subjects (268). This was followed up by similar results in a subsequent, similar study that found significantly reduced endogenous PKA activity and [3H] cAMP binding sites in the PFC of depressed suicide victims (269). Another study of suicide subjects noted a significant decrease in CRE-DNA binding activity, CREB messenger RNA and protein levels in the hippocampus and Broadmann area 9 of the brain, which includes part of the pre-frontal cortex, when compared to non-psychiatric healthy control subjects (270). These findings were also partially supported by that from a subsequent study of teenage suicide victims, which noted a decrease in CRE-DNA binding activity, CREB messenger RNA and protein expression in the PFC of suicide victims relative to healthy controls (271, 272). However, this study found no changes in the protein or messenger RNA expression of CREB in the hippocampus region of the suicide victims' brains, contradicting the findings of the study mentioned previously.

Overall, signal transduction abnormalities based on PKA, PKC and CREB findings have been implicated in suicidal behaviour. This is a promising area of research, part of the broader goal of identifying biological risk factors associated with suicidal behaviour that may be relevant to future therapeutic interventions (273). We are unaware of any studies to date that have investigated the role of these signal transduction pathways in the aetiology of NSSI.

4.7   Neuro-Inflammation

Growing evidence has emerged in recent years that inflammation may be an important factor in the pathophysiology of both major depression and suicidal behaviour. Studies have linked suicidal behaviour with a range of pro-inflammatory cytokines including interleukins 2, 6, 8 (IL-2, IL-6, IL-8 respectively) and tumour necrosis factor alpha (TNF-α).

Inflammatory markers (TNF-α, IL-6, IL-10 and C-reactive protein) have been shown to be significantly higher in patients with major depressive disorder (MDD) and high suicidal ideation, relative to those with MDD but lower suicidal ideation (274). There was no significant difference in the inflammatory index between those with MDD plus low suicidal ideation and those subjects in the non-depressed control group. Further analysis showed that the differences shown between MDD patients with high and low suicidal ideation were independent of depression severity and recent histories of suicide attempts, suggesting that the relationship between inflammation and suicidal ideation may be independent in depressed patients. This is supported by the conclusion of a systematic review, stating that changes in the inflammatory cytokine profile in subjects with major depressive disorder (MDD) depend on whether suicidal ideation or suicide attempts are present (275).

The review also acknowledged that evidence for associations between inflammatory cytokines and suicidal behaviour is not always consistently positive. A subsequent and the latest review in this area have highlighted an overall paucity of data available (276). Most studies have been cross-sectional and longitudinal data is needed to establish the role inflammation plays in the pathophysiology of suicidal behaviour in the long-term. In summary, based on the literature available, pro-inflammatory markers including interferons alpha and gamma (IFN-α, IFN-γ respectively), IL-1, IL-6 and TNF-α have been shown to be elevated in suicide attempters and victims versus normal controls. IL-6 in particular has been shown to be elevated not only in the cerebrospinal fluid but also in the peripheral blood of suicide attempters, showing promise as a possible biological suicide marker (276).

4.8   Neuro-Imaging Findings

In recent years, technological developments has allowed the increasing use of neuroimaging techniques such as functional magnetic resonance imaging (fMRI) and diffusion tensor imaging (DTI) to explore potential structural and functional abnormalities in the brains of individuals who engage in self-harm. Like other areas of research regarding the neurobiology underlying self-harm, the majority of studies have focused on suicidal behaviour in particular. However, a handful of studies have found structural and functional abnormalities in the brains of patients with NSSI as well. The participants in most of these NSSI studies had a diagnosis of borderline personality disorder (BPD), as self-harm is common and estimated to occur in 50 – 80% of BPD patients (258). A review on neuroimaging and NSSI concluded that there is little evidence for structural abnormalities in the brain of NSSI subjects but evidence from fMRI studies indicate possible functional abnormalities in the form of hyperactivity in the limbic structures of patients with NSSI and BPD (197).

Other reviews have been done on neuroimaging and suicidal behaviour or more precisely a history of suicidal attempts. Orbitofrontal cortex dysfunction (linked to the preference of options with high immediate reward) and reduced activity of the dorsolateral pre-frontal cortex have both been implicated in suicidal behaviour (277).

More recently, the first meta-analysis of imaging studies related to suicidal behaviour was published, which analysed studies with subjects with a psychiatric disorder plus a history of suicide attempts compared with subjects with only the psychiatric disorder and no history of suicide attempts (278). The results of the meta-analysis identified 6 regions of the brain, where structural or functional abnormalities were associated with a history of suicidal behaviour. For structural abnormalities characterised by a decreased volume of that region of the brain, the regions implicated were the left superior temporal and rectal gyri, as well as the caudate nucleus. For functional abnormalities characterised by hyper-reactivity to emotional stimuli and hypo-reactivity to cognitive stimuli, the regions implicated were the anterior and posterior parts of the right cingulate gyrus. Broadly speaking, the structurally abnormal areas implicated are involved in the processing of negative emotions. Taken with the functionally abnormal areas involved in the regulation of responses to emotional stimuli, these findings suggest a link between suicidal behaviour and the altered processing of negative emotions, leading to the negative stimuli being abnormally salient, and a reduced control over the intentional behavioural reaction to such stimuli (278).

Based on the few studies conducted on children and adolescents, the latest review noted that suicidal ideation was associated with reduced white matter in the orbitofrontal cortex (OFC) and an increased number of suicide attempts in adolescents was associated with reduced grey and white matter in the anterior cingulate (279). These findings support that of the aforementioned meta-analysis, suggesting that changes in the frontal systems involved with the processing of negative emotions play a role in the pathophysiology of suicidal behaviour. Structurally, the review noted that grey matter of the OFC is also typically reduced in suicide attempters, with the greater the decrease, the higher the lethality of the suicide attempt in borderline personality disorder (BPD) subjects. Functionally, some evidence indicates reduced blood flow to the PFC in response to word generation in suicide attempters, as well as reduced activity in the OFC in BPD suicide attempters. This is in line with the findings of a previous review (277). Since the OFC and PFC are both involved in the complicated processes behind human decision-making (280, 281), these findings would suggest that dysfunction in the cognitive processes behind decision-making is part of the pathophysiology of suicidal behaviour.

4.9   Summary

Our understanding of the neurobiology associated with self-harm and suicidal behaviour especially has grown significantly over the past few decades. The pathophysiology of self-harm and suicidal behaviour is complex and most likely involves a variety of neurobiological systems, ranging from the HPA axis to the endogenous opioid system and to neuro-inflammatory markers. Out of all this, the serotonergic system has been investigated the most thoroughly and a significant body of evidence supports the notion that dysfunction of this system is implicated in the pathophysiology of suicidality, independent of psychiatric co-morbidities. Some findings, such as low CSF 5-HIAA levels in suicide attempters versus healthy controls, have been replicated relatively consistently across studies. This contrasts with the lack of consistency in the limited data available for other areas, including that related to the HPA axis, noradrenergic and dopaminergic systems, as well as signal transduction pathways. The inconsistency and gaps in the data available in each of these areas have largely precluded any reasonably definitive conclusions about possible neurobiological mechanisms behind self-harm behaviour.

In addition, research into the neurobiological mechanisms behind NSSI has been very limited compared to that related to suicidal behaviour. In spite of this, research into the endogenous opioid system and pain perception has focused largely on NSSI instead of suicidal behaviour. It is reasonably clear that there is an imbalance in endogenous opioid levels and altered pain perception in individuals who engage in NSSI. While a functional model of NSSI behaviour has been put forward, further research is needed to validate the hypotheses drawn up.

The clinical relevance of neurobiological findings associated with self-harm remains to be seen. Nevertheless, there is a great deal of potential in the field to inform future therapeutic interventions. It may also be possible to generate useful biological markers for screening and clinical assessment purposes in the future. Overall, the field of neurobiology and self-harm behaviour is growing and may be of value in the future in improving our understanding of the pathophysiology and aetiology of self-harm.

5

Effective Interventions for Self-Harm

It is well established that self-harm is a major risk factor of suicide, increasing the risk of subsequent suicide by up to ten-fold (83). An estimated one in 25 patients who present to hospital with an episode of self-harm will die of suicide in the following 5 years (282) and approximately 15% of those who go on to die of suicide would have presented to a hospital emergency department in the year before death (283). In recent years, although the risk of suicide remains a major factor for consideration when treating this group of patients, research has highlighted a variety of other elevated risks associated with self-harm. These risks include alcohol misuse (284), psychiatric co-morbid diagnoses ranging from depression to conduct disorder in adolescents (285), as well as poorer educational and employment outcomes for those who engage in self-harm (82).

Suicide prevention strategies can traditionally be divided into population-based strategies and intervention-based strategies, with the former aimed at large, general population groups and the latter aimed at smaller, more specific high-risk groups. Population-based strategies that have demonstrated some success include the introduction of media guidelines for judicious reporting of suicides (286), gatekeeper training (287) and psychoeducation (288). Another successful population-based strategy is the restriction of access to means of suicide, which is widely used in many countries worldwide. It has been shown to be effective in reducing suicides (289) and is particularly effective when the restricted method is highly lethal and widely available (290).

It is clear that population-based strategies alone are insufficient and it is crucial that intervention-based strategies targeting high-risk individuals are implemented alongside. Adolescents and young adults represent a particularly vulnerable age group, as suicide is the second leading cause of the death for them (95).

For the purpose of this chapter, where possible, only randomised controlled trials (RCTs) focusing specifically on therapeutic interventions aiming to reduce self-harm (defined broadly as that with or without suicidal intent) in adolescents will be reviewed in detail. Research into therapeutic interventions for reducing self-harm in adolescents is largely based on a wide range of psychotherapies, as no pharmacological intervention has been shown to reduce self-harm behaviour in adolescents effectively and no RCTs investigating the effect of a specific pharmacological intervention for the reduction of self-harm in adolescents have been published.

5.1   Developmental Group Psychotherapy

Developmental group psychotherapy (DGP) is a type of group therapy specifically designed for adolescents who engage in self-harm. Combining techniques from a variety of other psychotherapeutic interventions, including dialectical behaviour therapy (DBT) and psychodynamic group psychotherapy (291), DGP can be considered to have three phases. After the initial assessment phase, there is a second phase consisting of 6 "acute" group sessions, before the third phase of weekly group therapy sessions in a "long-term" group, which can continue indefinitely as the individual sees fit.

DGP was first studied in 2001 in Manchester, England, via a single-blind, pilot, randomised controlled trial of 63 adolescents (291). The adolescents (aged 12 – 16 years, mean age 14, 78% female, deliberately self-harmed irrespective of intent on at least 2 occasions within past year) were randomly allocated to DGP on top of routine care or routine care alone. The primary outcomes, depression and suicidal behaviour, were assessed by direct interview at 29 weeks follow-up on average. Intention-to-treat analyses showed that adolescents part of the DGP group tended to have significantly fewer further self-harm episodes by the end of the study compared to those who were part of the routine care only group (6% in DGP group vs. 32% in routine care only group). For those adolescents who had a further episode of self-harm during the study, those in the DGP group tended to have their first repeat episode significantly later (11.9

weeks in DGP group vs. 7 weeks in routine care only group), and have fewer repeat episodes overall than those in the routine care only group. The DGP intervention had no significant effect on depressive symptoms or suicidal ideation.

This study is notable for many reasons. It was the first RCT ever to demonstrate that a psychological intervention has a statistically significant effect in adolescents who self-harm. We have highlighted the strengths and limitations of the study in Table 5.1 below. It is also clear from this study that unlike a widely made assumption at the time, therapeutic interventions targeting adolescents in groups may be beneficial instead of doing more harm than good.

Strengths of Study	Limitations of Study
Relatively good engagement with treatments, low refusal rate (16 out of 80 eligible subjects refused)	Relatively small sample size, leading to wide confidence intervals for effect size
Well-characterised randomisation and treatment allocation concealment	The amount of routine care given to adolescents were not controlled (possible confounding factor)
Intention-to-treat analyses conducted	No data on the cost-effectiveness of intervention
Outcome data available for 98% of adolescents	Some outcomes based on self-report
Reported range of outcomes related to subject's wellbeing in addition to primary outcomes	Relatively brief follow-up, so long-term effects of intervention unknown
Broad inclusion criteria, allowing sample to be more representative of that seen in routine clinical care and allowing results to be more generalisable as a result	Poor applicability likely in other settings
Only two therapists was required to administer the intervention	Unclear what and how much training required to administer intervention

Table 5.1: Strengths and Limitations of the Original Developmental Group Psychotherapy (DGP) Study (291).

Following the encouraging results from this initial pilot study on DGP, a slightly larger single-bind, randomised controlled trial was conducted in three sites in Australia (292), in an attempt to replicate and validate the findings notedin Manchester. 72 adolescents (aged 12 – 16 years, mean age 14, 91% female, deliberately self-harmed irrespective of intent on at least 2 occasions within past year) were randomly allocated to DGP on top of routine care or routine care alone. Unlike the original DGP study, the primary outcome for this replication study did not include depression or suicidal behaviour, but was focused on repetition of self-harm, which was assessed after 6 and 12 months follow-up on average. Like the original study, a range of secondary outcome measures was reported, including suicidal ideation, disruptive behaviour and service use. This study failed to replicate the promising results of the original study. It found that a higher number of adolescents in the DGP intervention group than those in the routine care only group had self-harmed by 6 months follow-up (88.2% in DGP group vs. 67.7% in routine care only group, p=0.04). Similar results were found for the follow-up period of 6 to 12 months, with more adolescents in the intervention group engaging in self-harm than that in the routine care group - although for this particular time period, the results were statistically non-significant (88.2% in DGP group vs. 67.7% in routine care only group, p=0.07).

Whilst the original study found that a lower proportion of adolescents in the DGP intervention group versus that in the routine care only group engaged in at least one episode of self-harm during the follow-up period of the study, this replication study found no statistically significant differences in the proportion of repeated self-harmers between the groups after 6 months (65% in DGP group vs. 53% in routine care only group, p=0.32). For the follow-up period of 6 to 12 months, a statistically non-significant trend was noted, where a greater proportion of adolescents in the DGP group repeated self-harm than that in the routine care only group (76% in DGP group vs. 56% in routine care only group, p=0.07). In addition, few differences were noted between the two arms of the trial for secondary outcome measures. Like the original study, the DGP intervention had no statistically significant effect on depressive symptoms or suicidal ideation.

Although this replication study failed to replicate the promising results of the original study, there were several key limitations of this replication study and differences between the two studies. One limitation was its smaller-than-anticipated sample size, which only reached 57% of the study's recruitment target to provide 80% power for the detection of moderate-sized treatment effects. The researchers acknowledged that the results seen could have been due to a failed trial, rather than a trial with negative findings. However, the smaller original study still had enough statistical power to detect the statistically significant treatment effect that it did. Other possible limitations include the fact that unlike the British therapists, the Australian therapists were not involved in the original development of the DGP intervention. Despite the training and supervision they received, the Australian therapists may not have strictly adhered to the original intervention program and could have lacked experience in delivering the intervention itself.

The sample characteristics of the replication study also differed from that of the original study. Compared to the British sample of the original study, a greater proportion of the Australian participants were female. Australian participants also tended to attend more counselling sessions overall (regardless of treatment allocation) and to engage in further episodes of self-harm during the follow-up period compared to their British counterparts. These differences in participant characteristics may have accounted for the different outcomes found in the replication study.

Following the replication study, another study was subsequently completed to re-examine the effectiveness of DGP intervention for self-harm in young people (293). The single-blind study design was identical to that of the previous two studies, with randomised allocation to DGP on top of routine care or routine care only, but this study was substantially larger in sample size and based at multiple sites in Northwest England. 366 adolescents in total (aged 12 – 17 years, 88.5% female, deliberately self-harmed irrespective of intent on at least 2 occasions within past year) were randomly allocated to DGP on top of routine care or routine care alone. The study found no significant differences in the frequency of subsequent self-harm episodes (OR = 0.99, 95% CI = 0.68 – 1.44, p = 0.95), the severity of those self-harm episodes at 1 year follow-up (OR = 0.81, 95% CI = 0.54 – 1.20, p = 0.29) and in the per-person cost required at 1 year follow-up when comparing the DGP intervention with the routine care only arm

(£21,781 for DGP group vs. £15,372 for routine care only group, p = 0.132). There were no significant differences between the two trial arms for secondary outcomes, including mood, suicidal ideation and health service use, although overall the whole cohort (regardless of treatment allocation) improved significantly from baseline.

The results of this latest study on DGP contradict that of the original pilot study but are in line with the Australian replication study. Some of the key strengths and limitations of this latest study are detailed in Table 5.2 below.

Strengths of Study	Limitations of Study
Large sample size – one of the largest RCTs ever on self-harm in adolescents	Unclear as to why there was an overall improvement for the whole cohort – possible regression to the mean, natural history of adolescent self-harm, or due to considerable routine care given?
Well-characterised randomisation and treatment allocation concealment	Significant proportion of sample was receiving considerable ongoing help (77% had extensive use of general practitioner and > 20% had contact with community psychiatric nurse) – this level of ongoing, routine help may not be applicable to other geographical settings
Low attrition/drop-out rate < 4%	

Table 5.2: Strengths and Limitations of the Most Recent Developmental Group Psychotherapy (DGP) Study (293).

The participants part of this latest DGP study, as well as those part of the Australian replication study, tended to have higher baseline severity, complexity and chronicity of self-harm than those part of the original pilot study. A significant proportion (86%) of the cohort of this latest study continued to frequently use Child and Adolescent Mental Health Services (CAMHS) in the year of follow-up. The significant amount of ongoing help that adolescents in this latest study received may help to explain, at least in part, the overall improvement seen in the entire cohort during the study from baseline to follow-up. The conclusion of this latest DGP study is that the addition of DGP does not appear to be cost-effective, or effective at improving self-harm outcomes in adolescents with repeated self-harm episodes. The possible reasons behind the considerable improvement made by the whole cohort should be examined in further detail. Further follow-up of this well-characterised cohort in the future could provide useful insight into the natural history of repetitive self-harm in adolescents and into the effects of different health service usage on this population group.

5.2   Multi-Systemic Therapy (MST) and Family Interventions

Another type of psychotherapy that has been used to treat self-harm in adolescents is multi-systemic therapy (MST). As its name suggests, MST targets the multiple systems a given young individual is part of, from family to community systems, as well as school and peer systems. MST can be viewed as a modified version of family therapy. It is a home-based, family-centered, intensive (daily contact may be required) but time limited (typically 3-5 months) intervention, aimed at developing effective parenting skills that focus on engaging the young individual in social rather than anti-social activities.

A randomised controlled trial (RCT) has investigated the effects of MST on self-harm behaviour in adolescents. The study focused on aspects of suicidal behaviour as outcome measures instead of self-harm episodes irrespective of intent. The aim of the study was to evaluate the efficacy of MST in reducing suicide attempts in adolescents who were referred and approved for emergency psychiatric hospitalisation in South Carolina, USA (294). Of the 156 adolescents (aged 10 – 17 years, mean age 12.9 years, 65% male, 65% African American, predominantly from low socioeconomic backgrounds), 51% were deemed "suicidal" due to the presence of suicidal ideation, plan or attempt. The adolescents were randomly allocated to MST or hospitalisation and followed up for 1 year post-treatment. Based on youth reports, MST was significantly more effective at reducing rates of suicide attempts at 1-year follow-up and appeared to provide faster symptom relief than hospitalisation. However, MST did not have a significantly different effect on hopelessness, suicidal ideation or depression compared to that observed in the hospitalisation group. Taking into account the strengths and limitations of this study presented in Table 5.3, the findings of this study were generally positive and in support of MST as an effective therapeutic intervention for adolescents who engage in suicide attempts.

Strengths of Study	Limitations of Study
Rare and under-researched sample group – predominantly low socioeconomic and ethnic minority background	Sample may not be very generalizable - its composition being predominantly African-American, from low-income family backgrounds and presenting to hospital with psychiatric emergency
Well-characterised randomisation and treatment allocation concealment	Mean age of sample unusually young for studies of adolescents with self-harm and self-harm was presenting problem for only a minority of sample
Low attrition/drop-out rate of 2.5%, 74/79 families completed full course of MST intervention for an average of 127 days	Youths in the intervention group had significantly higher rates of suicide attempts prior to treatment than those in hospitalisation group – so the positive effects of the intervention may reflect a regression to the mean effect instead of a truly positive effect of the intervention
Use of validated measures of suicidal behaviour and suicidal ideation	Rates of attempted suicide fell in both intervention and hospitalisation groups over the year of follow-up so the significant decline in symptoms in those part of the intervention group may represent the natural history of suicide attempts in youths
	Applicability issues: Intervention requires substantial resources and training often not available in community child psychiatric services

Table 5.3: Strengths and Limitations of the Multi-Systemic Therapy (MST) Study (294)

Following the publication of the results of the MST study, a brief report was published soon after (295) focusing specifically on the 70 adolescents who took part in the MST study and who engaged in self-harm behaviour prior to being referred to the hospital. The aim of this report was to analyse the factors that may predict poor treatment response in the sample of 70 adolescents. As part of the study, the 70 adolescents (aged 10 – 17 years, mean age 13.4 years, standard deviation = 2.2, 60% male, 67% African American, 33% European American) were randomly allocated to either MST or inpatient psychiatric hospitalization. After completing their treatment, the report divided the youths into "treatment responders" or "treatment non-responders" depending on reports of suicide attempts given by the youth or caregivers. Correlations were found between youth suicide attempts and female gender, depressive affect, youth-rated parental control, caregiver psychiatric hospitalisation history as well as caregiver psychiatric distress. However, out of all these correlates, the only independent factors that predicted treatment non-response in youths were depressive affect and youth-rated parental control. These findings suggest that adaptations to MST may need to be considered to address some risk factors in youths not responding to treatment, and in particular to address depression in youths with self-harm using additional therapeutic interventions.

In addition to the MST study, other randomised trials have investigated the effects of home-based family interventions in adolescents with self-harm, although results have been less promising than that found in the MST study. An RCT investigated the effects of a home-based family intervention delivered by child psychiatric social workers on children and adolescents who have deliberately poisoned themselves (296). The intervention involved one assessment session followed by 4 home visits by social workers to run family problem-solving sessions. The RCT included 162 patients (age ≤ 16 years) who were randomly allocated to routine care only (n = 77, received no home visits) or routine care plus intervention (n = 85). The primary outcomes, namely suicidal ideation as assessed by the Suicidal Ideation Questionnaire, hopelessness as assessed by the Hopelessness Scale and family functioning as assessed by the Family Assessment Device, were assessed at 2 and 6 months follow-up after recruitment. There were no significant differences between the intervention and the control groups for any of the primary outcomes at 2 and 6 months follow-up. However, a subgroup of participants without major depression in the intervention group was noted to have significantly reduced suicidal ideation at 2 and 6 months follow-up compared to those in the control group, indicating that the family-based intervention may only benefit those without major depression.

The same research group who conducted the trial then went on to do further analysis (297) of the data from the trial to examine the possible reasons behind the different responses to the brief family intervention from depressed and non-depressed young people. They found that the reduction in suicidal ideation observed in non-depressed young people part of the intervention group was not mediated by changes in variables including compliance with treatment and changes in family functioning. It was therefore postulated that since those young people who were depressed had more suicidal ideation and hopelessness than those who were non-depressed, the family intervention may have been too brief to have significant effects on those with major depression. Further research into more intensive and lengthier forms of family intervention may be warranted in the future to target young people with major depression who engage in self-harm.

A cost-effectiveness analysis (298) was also conducted for this family intervention study and it found no significant differences in the costs involved for the intervention group relative to that for the control group.

Another RCT (299) investigated the efficacy of a social support-based intervention called the Youth Nominated Support Team – Version II (YST-II), on top of routine care for 448 psychiatrically hospitalised, suicidal adolescents (aged 13 – 17 years, mean age 15.59, 71.2% female, 84% Caucasian, significant suicidal ideation or suicide attempt in past four weeks). Following psychiatric hospitalisation, the adolescents were randomised into the treatment as usual plus YST-II intervention group, or the TAU only group, which acted as the control. The YST-II intervention consists of psychoeducation and consultations for the adults that have been nominated by the youths themselves as their support person. In turn, the support person maintains regular contact with and provides support to the adolescent for 3 months post-hospitalisation. As part of the YST-II intervention, adolescents selected an average of 3.43 (SD = 0.83) people as their nominated support adults. Outcome measures of the trial included suicidal ideation, depression, hopelessness, functional impairment, alcohol or substance use disorders if applicable and suicide attempts. It was found that the YST-II intervention on top of routine care had very limited benefits in the form of a more rapid decline in suicidal ideation for those with a history of multiple suicide attempts during the first 6 weeks post-hospitalisation and in functional impairment at 3 and 12 months follow-up for non-multiple suicide attempters. However, the overall decline in suicidal ideation did not differ between the intervention and control groups and notably, the YST-II intervention had no impact on subsequent suicide attempts. No harmful effects of the intervention were observed.

Although these findings suggest only limited benefits of the YST-II intervention, they represent significant improvements compared to the findings of a previous trial that investigated the efficacy of the first version of the Youth-Nominated Support Team (YST-I) intervention in suicidal, psychiatrically hospitalised adolescents (300). In that trial, YST-I had no effects on suicide attempts, suicidal ideation or functional impairment. Compared to YST-I, the YST-II intervention only differed by the use of updated psychoeducation resources for support persons, allowing only adults and not peers to be support persons, and shortening the intervention period from 6 months to 3 months. In particular, the intervention period was shortened because in the first trial, between the third and six month of the intervention period, a 7-fold increase in the percentage of youths not contacted regularly was observed. Although the YST-II intervention is a feasible, non-intensive and relatively cheap supplemental intervention on top of routine care for suicidal adolescents, its benefits at the moment are too small to be consistent with recommending its widespread incorporation into clinical practice. Further research into YST-II or other similar multi-faceted, psychoeducational, social support- based intervention for suicidal adolescents is warranted.

5.3   Dialectical Behaviour Therapy (DBT)

Another type of intensive therapeutic intervention that has been used to reduce self-harm behaviours in young people is dialectical behaviour therapy (DBT). Originally developed to treat suicidality, DBT is a cognitive behavioural-based intervention comprising an intense schedule of individual therapy sessions every week, one group skills training session weekly, plus a therapist consultation team meeting. Traditionally, a significant proportion of research investigating the therapeutic effects of DBT was conducted in parasuicidal adult women with borderline personality disorder (BPD) and this area is hence one where the strongest evidence exists in support of the therapeutic effects of DBT (301). In recent years, DBT research has expanded to include adolescents with or without BPD, as well as young adults aged 18 – 25 without BPD.

DBT in adolescents uses a modified version of DBT, called DBT-A. It differs from original DBT in 5 key aspects presented in Table 5.4. This adapted version of DBT was used in a study of suicidal adolescents with borderline personality symptoms (302). This quasi-experimental study was not a RCT, with imbalanced groups (n = 29 in DBT-A group which had more severe pre-treatment symptoms than the treatment as usual TAU

group, n = 82) but did find that the 12-week DBT-A reduced suicidal ideation and general psychiatric symptoms including symptoms of border-line
personality disorder. Compared to the TAU group, the DBT-A group also
had significant reduced rates of psychiatric hospitalisations during the
treatment period and a significantly higher rate of treatment completion.
The latter finding is of clinical relevance, as poor engagement with therapy
is a common and key barrier to achieving desired clinical outcomes from
treatment of suicidal or self-harm behaviour in adolescents.

Original DBT	DBT-A	Reason for Modification in DBT-A
Typically can last up to 1 year	Intervention period shortened, often down to 12 weeks	Shorter time period more realistic for adolescent engagement and comple-tion of therapy
Family members of individual not included in weekly skills training group session	Family members of in-dividual included in weekly skills training group session	To educate family members who can then serve as coaches and to improve the often dysfunctional home envi-ronment of adolescent
Individual one-to-one therapy sessions	Including family mem-bers when discussing familial issues in indi-vidual therapy sessions	To improve familial relationships and home environment of adolescent
Standard hand-outs and a wide range of skills taught during DBT course	Simplified language used in handouts and a reduced range of skills taught	To maximise the skills learnt and maintained by adolescents as part of the 12 week course
No "Walking the Mid-dle Path" Skills Module	"Walking the Middle Path" Skills Module aimed at adolescents and their families (303)	Additional skills module with particu-lar emphasis on the often problematic or stressful relationship between the adolescent and their family

Table 5.4: Modifications of Dialectical Behaviour Therapy (DBT) for Adolescents (DBT-A).

Since these two RCTs supporting the acceptability and feasibility of
implementing DBT as a therapeutic intervention for adolescents who engage in self-harm behaviour, the latest and largest RCT to date aimed to

investigate the clinical efficacy of DBT-A at reducing self-harm in adolescents (309). This RCT studied the effects of 19-weeks of DBT-A in a sample of 77 adolescents (88.3% female) with recent and repetitive self-harm relative to the effects of enhanced usual care (EUC). EUC consisted of 19 weeks of standard care, only "enhanced" by the criterion that EUC therapists provide at least one weekly treatment session per patient throughout the study. Like that found in the pilot study, treatment retention was relatively good (74.4% in DBT-A group). In this RCT, no significant differences in treatment engagement were found between the DBT-A and the EUC groups. However, DBT-A was shown to be significantly better at reducing self-harm episodes, severity of suicidal ideation and depressive symptoms in adolescents relative to EUC, as assessed at 9, 15 and 19 weeks.

Most of the studies on DBT focus on suicidal behaviour but some have started to investigate the effects of DBT on NSSI specifically, separating NSSI outcomes with the outcome of self-harm in general with or without suicidal intent. For example, a recent pilot study of a community-based, 26-week long DBT programme in 6 female, suicidal adolescents found a self-reported decrease in suicidality and NSSI events, in addition to an improvement in emotion regulation at 3-months follow-up (310). Moreover, the latest systematic review of the different treatments available for NSSI identified 4 RCTs that investigated the effect of DBT on NSSI outcomes (311). The findings of the 4 RCTs are mixed, with two of them finding that DBT reduces NSSI relative to routine treatment and the other two finding that the effects of DBT on NSSI is comparable to routine treatment. Although one of the trials that found a beneficial effect of DBT on reducing NSSI frequency used a sample of young adult college students aged 18 – 25, none of the 4 RCTs included adolescents aged below 18 in their samples. Overall, it remains unclear as to whether DBT has any specific therapeutic benefits on NSSI outcomes in adolescents.

Nevertheless, the DBT studies done using adult samples have noted a range of beneficial effects of DBT on aspects of suicidal and self-harm behaviour. The therapeutic effects of DBT that have been observed in these studies include a reduction of NSSI episodes (312), suicide attempts (312, 313), depressive symptoms and psychiatric medication use (314), hospitalisation for suicidal ideation or psychiatric emergencies (313), aggression and irritability (315), as well as improvements in emotion regulation (316) and treatment engagement (313).

These findings in adults are promising and indicate that it is worthwhile to continue further research to investigate if similar beneficial effects can be translated to adolescent samples. In a relatively recent systematic review of the clinical efficacy of DBT for suicidal adolescents aged 18 or younger (317), all studies included in the review reported DBT as having a certain degree of efficacy in reducing suicidality, self-harm and suicide ideation in adolescents. This area of research is continuing to grow in both inpatient (318) and in community-based programmes (310). Future studies should aim to study the effects of DBT in larger samples of adolescents and include longer-term follow-up evaluations to monitor the maintenance of any improvements in self-harm outcomes observed.

5.4   Interpersonal Psychotherapy (IPT)

Interpersonal psychotherapy (IPT) is a time-limited intervention of weekly therapy sessions typically lasting a total of 12 to 16 weeks. Briefly, the format of IPT is as follows - a target diagnosis such as major depressive disorder is identified, then the IPT therapist links the diagnosis to interpersonal problems, and the therapist supports the patient to focus on solving the interpersonal problems and learn interpersonal skills along the way, improving the symptoms of the target diagnosis identified (319). IPT has been well established as an effective psychotherapeutic intervention for depression in adolescents (320), improving overall functioning and reducing depressive symptoms better than treatment as usual (321). Evidence also suggests that adolescents engage with IPT treatment relatively well (322). However, the effects of IPT on self-harm or suicidal behaviour in depressed adolescents have largely been unexplored. Only one relevant RCT has been identified, where a sample of 73 depressed adolescents with suicidal risk were randomised to either the intensive interpersonal psychotherapy for adolescents with suicidal risk (IPT-A-IN) group or the treatment as usual group (323). Those in the IPT-A-IN group had lower severity of depression, suicidal ideation, anxiety and hopelessness post-intervention relative to those in the treatment as usual group, indicating that intensive IPT may be effective at reducing overall suicidal risk in high-risk, depressed adolescents. These findings have yet to be independently replicated, but do support IPT as a potential suicide prevention strategy in depressed adolescents.

5.5   Cognitive Behavioural Therapy (CBT)

Like IPT, cognitive behavioural therapy (CBT) is a well-established psychotherapeutic intervention for the treatment of depression in adolescents (324). The number of CBT efficacy studies in depressed adolescents has increased over the past decade, but it remains unclear whether the efficacy of CBT in treating depression in adolescents extends to clinically relevant benefits for suicidal behaviour or self-harm outcomes (325).

One early RCT investigated the effects of a cognitively oriented therapy called LifeSPAN therapy in addition to standard care in 56 suicidal young people aged 15 – 25, having experienced their first episode of psychosis (326). Compared to the control group that received standard care only, the LifeSPAN group demonstrated a larger mean decrease in suicidal ideation, hopelessness and a larger improvement in quality of life. The majority of RCTs in this area of research have used proxy measures that have well-established links to suicidal behaviour, such as hopelessness.

Larger RCTs have subsequently been conducted, including one called the Treatment for Adolescents with Depression Study (TADS). The TADS trial was a multicentre, large RCT that investigated the effects of combining CBT with anti-depressant medication (fluoxetine), relative to fluoxetine alone or CBT alone in 327 adolescents aged 12 – 17 years with major depressive disorder (327). With intention-to-treat analyses, it was found that combining CBT with fluoxetine had the highest rate of clinical response (as assessed by the Children's Depression Rating Scale-Revised) of the three groups at weeks 12, 18 and 36. Suicidal ideation decreased in all three groups, but more so in the CBT only and the combination of CBT and fluoxetine group. CBT also appeared to have a positive effect of reducing suicidal events (14.7%, 8.4%, 6.3% in fluoxetine only, combination and CBT only groups respectively).

Following the TADS study, a slightly smaller RCT called the Adolescent Depression Antidepressants and Psychotherapy Trial (ADAPT) was conducted consisting of 208 depressed adolescents aged 11 – 17 years, who have not responded to a brief initial psychosocial intervention by the Child and Adolescent Mental Health Services (328). The participants were randomised to routine care plus a selective serotonin-reuptake inhibitor (SSRI), or routine care plus SSRI and CBT. The evidence supporting CBT from the ADAPT trial was not as promising as that observed in the TADS study. From clinical characteristics, it was evident that the participants of the ADAPT trial as a whole were severely depressed. No significant differences in clinical outcomes, protection against adverse effects or cost-effectiveness were found with the addition of CBT to fluoxetine and routine care. The SSRI plus CBT interventions did not have any measurable effects on disinhibition, irritability and violence compared to levels at baseline. Approximately 20% of the patients in the trial were classed as non-responders as well, some of which showed no improvement by 28 weeks (43%) and some were even considered worse off (57%). In addition, both suicidal and non-suicidal self-harm persisted despite treatments provided as part of the ADAPT study (329).

A subsequent, larger RCT called the Treatment of Selective Serotonin Re-Uptake Inhibitor- Resistant Depression in Adolescents (TORDIA) study found similarly insignificant effects of CBT on outcomes including suicidal ideation, depression, hopelessness and self-reported anxiety in depressed adolescents (330). The sample consisted of 334 adolescents aged 12 – 18 years with a diagnosis of major depressive disorder or dysthymia that was resistant to 8 or more weeks of SSRI treatment, of which the SSRI dosage must be equivalent to at least 40mg of fluoxetine for the last 4 weeks of treatment. The adolescents were randomised to a medication swap only group or a medication swap plus CBT group. The rate of and time to remission, the rate of and time to relapse and the rate of adverse events were all similar for the CBT plus medication swap group versus the medication swap only group. Nonetheless, those in the CBT plus medication swap group showed a higher clinical response rate than those in the medication swap only group (54.8% vs. 40.5%, p = 0.009), as measured by the Clinical Global Impressions-Improvement Score and the Children's Depression Rating Scale-Revised (331). Outcomes were measured up to 24 weeks follow-up, making this study particularly useful in examining the short and long-term effects of CBT on depression and suicidal ideation in depressed adolescents.

Overall, evidence supporting the use of CBT to reduce suicidal or self-harm behaviour in adolescents is lacking. A rare systematic review looking at this topic noted a paucity of relevant studies available, and that whilst evidence supports the use of CBT in ameliorating suicidal behaviour in adults, the same cannot be said for adolescents (332). Combined with evidence of publication bias, the evidence supporting CBT as a therapeutic intervention for self-harm in adolescents remains too inconsistent and limited to recommend the incorporation of CBT into routine clinical practice for adolescents who engage in self-harm.

Nevertheless, researchers have continued to explore CBT-based interventions for self-harm. One such intervention is called manual-assisted cognitive therapy (MACT), which is a brief intervention consisting of 6 sessions of focused therapy aiming to help patients improve their understanding of self-harm behaviour and problem-solve. Manuals guide the therapy sessions and cover a range of topics including "Understanding self-harm" and "What to do in a crisis". A few RCTs have been conducted investigating the efficacy of MACT in reducing self-harm, although none have been conducted in adolescent only cohorts. Overall, evidence from the RCTs supports MACT as a feasible and effective intervention in reducing self-harm behaviour (333 – 336). More RCTs with larger sample sizes and strictly adolescent (aged 18 or below) cohorts are warranted in the future to explore this.

Another type of CBT intervention is one designed for suicidal adolescents with co-occurring alcohol or other drug disorder (AOD). Having shown to be feasible and acceptable as an integrated outpatient therapeutic intervention for such adolescents in a pilot study (337), a subsequent RCT used intention-to-treat analyses in a cohort of 40 adolescent psychiatric inpatients and demonstrated that this integrated CBT intervention was associated with a significantly reduced number of suicide attempts, psychiatric hospitalisations and emergency department presentations relative to that associated with enhanced treatment as usual (338). However, no significant differences in the degree of suicidal ideation reductions were observed between the two groups.

New adaptations of CBT-based interventions have recently emerged too, including computerised CBT (cCBT) and mindfulness-based cognitive therapy (MBCT). Preliminary evidence for cCBT has been supportive so far. It has been shown in a systematic review that cCBT can reduce clinical symptoms of depression and anxiety, and boost self-esteem and improve behaviour in children and adolescents (339). The first RCT investigating the efficacy of MCT in reducing NSSI in young people is also currently underway (340).

A novel cognitive-behavioural family intervention for suicidal adolescents called Safe Alternatives for Teens & Youths (SAFETY) has been developed recently as well, consisting of a 12-week CBT intervention designed to be integrated with emergency services and to focus specifically on reducing suicidal behaviour. Although no RCTs have been done yet investigating the efficacy of the SAFETY program, a preliminary treatment development trial has been conducted (341). 35 adolescents aged 11 – 18 years who had a recent history of suicide attempts in the past 3 months were enrolled on to the 12-week SAFETY program. Significant improvements in suicidal behaviour, hopelessness, youth and parent depression and youth social adjustment were observed at 3 months follow-up relative to baseline. Treatment satisfaction was noted to be high. These promising findings support the pursuit of a RCT to investigate and explore the feasibility and efficacy of the SAFETY intervention in suicidal adolescents at high risk of further suicidal behaviour.

5.6   Emergency Department Interventions

The emergency department (ED) is often a prime location to screen and identify adolescents at risk of self-harm or suicidal behaviour. A cross-sectional study of adolescent suicide attempters aged 13 – 19 years found that 82% visit an ED for any reason in the year prior to their suicide attempt, and of this group, 26% visit an ED for psychiatric reasons including suicidal ideation and self-harm (342). The ED therefore also represents an opportunity, albeit a brief one, to intervene and provide treatment for adolescents who engage in self-harm behaviour.

Since ED visits tend to be too brief to provide therapeutic interventions aiming to reduce self-harm behaviour in the long-term, ED-based therapeutic interventions mostly aim to improve adherence to subsequent outpatient treatment. Evidence from an early study (343) suggests that a specialised program of care in the ED (consisting of special training for ED staff to alter their behaviour and expectations when caring for suicide attempters and their families, a short 20 minute video for adolescent suicide attempters and their families to improve their understanding of adolescent suicidality and treatment, plus a brief family therapy session conducted by a crisis therapist in the emergency room) significantly improves attendance of the first outpatient treatment session (95.4% in specialised program group vs. 82.7% in routine care group) and of subsequent follow-up treatment sessions (5.7% in specialised program group vs. 4.7% in routine group). In addition, adolescent suicide attempters who were in the specialised program group reported fewer psychiatric symptoms and the mothers of those adolescents reported more positive attitudes toward treatment relative to the relevant counterparts in the routine emergency care group.

A long-term, 18-month follow-up of this specialised emergency room care intervention in the same cohort of 140 female adolescent suicide attempters aged 12 – 18 years noted that the intervention group was associated with significantly lower self-reported depression scores (344). The rate of subsequent suicide attempts following the initial one was lower than expected in both groups and was in fact too low to allow for any meaningful comparison between the two groups. Nevertheless, these findings indicate that ED-based interventions such as this specialised care program can have modest benefits for adolescent suicide attempters who present to emergency departments.

Another ED-based intervention called the Family Intervention for Suicide Prevention (FISP) has been developed. Specially designed for use in routine ED settings, FISP is a brief, focused, family-based CBT intervention that is partly based on the specialised emergency room intervention used in the aforementioned studies involving female adolescent suicide attempters. A RCT designed to investigate the efficacy of FISP relative to enhanced usual care (enhanced by education for the emergency care providers) in suicidal adolescents who present to ED with suicidal ideation or a suicide attempt was conducted. 181 adolescents aged 10 – 18 years participated and it was found that those randomised to the FISP intervention group had significantly higher rates relative to the control group of receiving outpatient treatment whether this was in the form of psychotherapy alone or combined with medication (345).

Other ED-based interventions have also been shown to help improve treatment engagement in adolescents who self-harm. For example, the Therapeutic Assessment intervention developed by Ougrin and colleagues as a manualised procedure able to be implemented in ED settings was shown in a RCT of adolescents who were newly referred to psychiatric services following an episode of self-harm to significantly improve the attendance of the first follow-up appointment and the likelihood of attending at least four subsequent treatment sessions (346). The 2-year follow-up of this RCT demonstrated that the positive effect of the Therapeutic Assessment intervention on treatment engagement was sustained (347).

The efficacy of another brief, ED-based intervention in improving subsequent treatment engagement and linkage to outpatient mental health services in adolescents who have been screened and identified as clinically at risk for suicide was examined in a pilot RCT (348). 24 adolescents aged 12 – 17 years screened positive for suicidal risk factors were randomised to the intervention package (consisting of a short motivational interview, barrier reduction, establishment of an outpatient appointment and reminders before the scheduled appointment) or standard referral (provision of a telephone number for a mental health provider) groups. Though the sample size was small, there was a significantly higher attendance of a subsequent mental health appointment during the follow-up period (63.6% in intervention group vs. 15.4% in standard referral group). A non-significant trend of a more significant improvement in depressive symptoms in the intervention group relative to the standard referral group was also noted.

In summary, the literature to date indicates that innovative ED-based interventions may be feasible and efficacious ways in improving outpatient treatment engagement for adolescents who engage in self-harm and may even have modest but clinically relevant effects in alleviating depressive symptoms.

5.7   Pharmacological Interventions

A range of pharmacological agents have been investigated over the years in the treatment of self-harm and suicide-related behaviour. They include selective serotonin re-uptake inhibitors (SSRIs), atypical anti-psychotics (e.g. clozapine), mood stabilisers (e.g. lamotrigine) and alpha-2 agonists (e.g. clonidine). A systematic review suggested that the aforementioned pharmacological agents may have some efficacy in the treatment of self-harm, although most of the evidence base in this area consists of open studies and clinical case reports (349). In this systematic review, the need for randomised, double-blind, placebo-controlled trials to be conducted were evident to substantiate the limited evidence available at the time to support the use of particular pharmacological agents for the treatment of self-harm.

There remain no randomised controlled trials investigating the efficacy of pharmacological interventions in the treatment of self-harm in adolescents (350). Some RCTs have however been conducted in adults who engage in self-harm. The latest systematic review of all RCTs including pharmacological agents or natural products for self-harm in adults found 7 trials with a total of 546 subjects (351). No significant treatment effects on the repetition of self-harm were noted for newer generation antidepressants (nomifensine, mianserin, paroxetine), low-dose fluphenazine, mood stabilisers or natural products (dietary supplementation of omega-3 fatty acids). Overall, the evidence available was of low or very low quality, and only a small number of relevant trials exist. Although one particular trial of the anti-psychotic flupenthixol was noted to have found a significant reduction in self-harm, this study was of very low quality according to the Grading of Recommendations, Assessment, Development and Evaluations (GRADE) criteria for appraising the quality of studies. Given that the evidence available is limited and generally of poor quality, this systematic review stated that no firm conclusions could be drawn about the effects of pharmacological interventions on self-harm outcomes in adults.

Focusing specifically on NSSI, only one RCT has been conducted evaluating the efficacy of a pharmacological intervention in reducing NSSI (311). This double-blind, placebo-controlled RCT was conducted in 52 adults (43 female, 9 male) with borderline personality disorder (352). The subjects were randomised to receive 15mg/day of aripiprazole or placebo for 8 weeks. Participants were followed up to 18 months (353). Using intention-to-treat analyses, significantly greater changes were observed in the intervention group relative to the placebo group for borderline personality symptoms, depression, anxiety and anger expression. Moreover, there was a reduction in NSSI behaviour observed in a greater proportion of participants in the intervention group than that in the placebo group. These findings have yet to be replicated independently.

An area of particular interest in child and adolescent psychiatry has been the use of anti-depressants (in particular, SSRIs) and their relation to self-harm. From the results of a robust meta-analysis of 372 double blind, placebo-controlled RCTs, the risk of suicidal behaviour associated with anti-depressants appeared to be age-dependent (354). Relative to the placebo groups, it appeared that there was an increased risk of suicidal behaviour among those less than 25 years old, a possibly neutral effect on suicidal behaviour for those aged 25 – 64 years old, and finally a reduced risk of suicidal behaviour in those aged 65 or above. This was supported by a review done in 2009 of evidence from RCTs, observational and ecological studies, which concluded that SSRIs are linked to an increased risk of suicide attempts in young people, but not in adults (355).

However, there is considerable controversy surrounding this association. Another review, albeit one of observational studies only, suggested that SSRIs are not associated with an increased risk of suicide in adolescents and it may be that those adolescents who die from suicide have not been on SSRIs long enough to benefit from the anti-depressant (356). This was supported by evidence from a large, retrospective, longitudinal cohort study of adolescents aged 12 – 18 years newly diagnosed with major depressive disorder (MDD), which found that antidepressant medication (whether this was SSRIs or another type of antidepressant) was not statistically significant in its association with the risk of suicide attempts (357).

Nevertheless, the Food and Drug Administration (FDA), the American organisation responsible for the regulation of medicines, made it compulsory in 2004 for SSRI manufacturers to have black boxes on their packaging with warnings of the increased risk of suicidality in pediatric patients. This has led to a change in antidepressant prescribing patterns for young people under the age of 18 years (358). There has been a decline in depression treatment using SSRIs after the FDA warnings were issued, which has persisted in both children and adult populations (359, 360). The FDA warnings have drawn considerable controversy and debate, with one large quasi-experimental study questioning whether the subsequent decrease in antidepressant use may actually be counterproductive and be linked to increases in suicide attempts in young people (361). However, many have questioned the quality of this study and remain unconvinced of the possible association between the FDA warning and an increase in suicide attempts in young people (362 – 366).

Looking beyond suicidal behaviour at the broader term of self-harm with or without the intent to die, using a propensity score matched cohort of 162,625 US residents with depression aged 10 – 64 years, it was found that young people aged 24 years or below who initiated antidepressant therapy with SSRIs at a high-therapeutic dose had an increased risk of self-harm (367). The increased risk was approximately twice that of matched patients who initiated SSRIs at a modal-dose (hazard ratio [HR] = 2.2, 95% CI = 1.6 – 3.0). The modal dose for citalopram hydrobromide, sertraline hydrochloride, and fluoxetine hydrochloride were 20 mg/day, 50 mg/day, and 20 mg/day respectively. Similar to studies mentioned previously, this increase in the risk of suicidal behaviour did not appear to affect adults aged 25 – 64 years nearly as much, and this cohort study found effectively no difference in risk between adults in that age range who started SSRIs at a high-therapeutic dose and those who started at a modal-dose.

A separate large cohort study of 238,963 patients aged 20 – 64 years newly diagnosed with depression observed that the rates of suicide, suicide attempts or self-harm were all similar regardless of which antidepressant class the patient was taking (368). Whilst these studies provide useful insights into the possible associations between antidepressant therapy and self-harm behaviour, few studies have focused specifically on adolescent populations. Since age, gender, pre-existing depression or suicidal ideations are all possible confounding factors that arise in many observational studies that examine the association between SSRIs and suicidal behaviour (369), large robust RCTs investigating the effects of antidepressants on specific self-harm outcomes in strictly adolescent samples are needed in the future.

5.8   Engagement with Therapy

No matter how effective a given psychotherapeutic intervention may be, desirable clinical outcomes can only be achieved if the young person engages with and remains compliant with the intervention. Adolescent suicide attempters have been known to tend to engage poorly with follow-up psychotherapy (370). A study of outpatient clinic attendance patterns of adolescents aged 10 – 18 years old found that high percentages (77%) drop out of treatment (371). It also noted that adolescent suicide attempters were more likely to miss more outpatient appointments and to drop out of treatment earlier than adolescent non-attempters. Another study of 71 adolescent suicide attempters found significant number disengage entirely (20% did not attend any follow-up appointments at all) or engage only briefly with follow-up treatment, with 39% having attended fewer than 3 sessions (372). Over 40% of a sample of 143 adolescent suicide attempters had their cases closed due to non-attendance of outpatient therapy sessions (373).

Since poor engagement with therapy has been demonstrated to be associated with poor outcomes including suicidal ideation and depressive symptoms in at-risk adolescents (374), some research has focused on exploring the range of factors that may predict or influence treatment compliance. These factors include parental attitudes (375, 376), age and gender of the adolescent, the presence or absence of vigorous case-tracking procedures (373), the degree of planning of the initial suicide attempt (377) as well as the severity of the adolescent's psychopathology (378). It is hoped that by understanding the factors that are associated with treatment compliance in adolescents who engage in self-harm, existing therapeutic interventions can be adapted or new therapeutic interventions developed to improve treatment engagement and hence improve the intervention's efficacy in helping adolescents achieve their desired outcomes.

Recently, a systematic review and meta-analysis of RCTs that investigated therapeutic interventions in adolescents who presented with self-harm was conducted (379). It found no statistically significant difference in the number of adolescents who failed to attend at least 4 sessions of treatment as usual (TAU) or specific psychological treatment (SPT). This meta-analysis has subsequently been updated (380) and the updated version found that the proportion of adolescents who failed to attend 4 or more sessions of SPT was in fact significantly lower than that for TAU (28.4% in SPT group vs. 45.9% in TAU group, p < 0.0001). This latest meta-analysis is the first to show that SPT not only reduces self-harm in adolescents but also improves adolescent engagement with treatment. One possible explanation for the different findings between this latest meta-analysis and its predecessor could be due to improvements in the available SPTs in recent years, making them more appealing for adolescents to engage with. However, only 12 studies were included in this meta-analysis, highlighting the fact that there remains a lack of good-quality, relevant RCTs in the field. Subgroup analyses were not conducted due to the small sample sizes used in the limited number of RCTs included in the meta-analysis. More research is therefore needed in the future to explore and characterise specific features of SPT that are associated with improved treatment compliance in adolescents who engage in self-harm.

5.9   Summary

Psychotherapeutic interventions are very much based on the skills of the person(s) who delivers the intervention and the proper delivery of such interventions will require training and supervision. Since self-harm and suicidal behaviour can have wide ranging underlying pathologies, it is also unrealistic to expect that any given type of psychotherapeutic intervention would meet the needs of every affected adolescent (381).

Currently, stronger evidence for the use of psychological interventions in the treatment of self-harm behaviour in adolescents exists than that for the use of pharmacological interventions. A range of psychotherapies have been investigated and in spite of occasionally conflicting results from different studies, most psychological interventions have shown some promise overall in reducing self-harm behaviour in adolescents (350). Independent replication of studies on DBT, MST and CBT are very much needed to substantiate some of the positive findings observed. Evidence also suggests that emergency department-based interventions are feasible and effective ways to promote outpatient follow-up treatment engagement for adolescents who engage in self-harm, which will be explored in greater detail in the next chapter.

To advance our knowledge of suicide prevention strategies, it is important for investigators in the field of suicide prevention to work with each other and with policymakers, to facilitate large-scale, multi-site cohort studies of high-risk groups and to facilitate the evaluation of suicide prevention programs respectively (382). Research aimed at reductions in youth suicide and suicidal behaviour via a public health approach, including increasing access to primary care-based interventions for at-risk youth and improving the continuity of care for those who present to emergency departments after a suicide attempt, is a particular priority with potentially far-reaching benefits (383). Effective upstream suicide prevention programs targeting children at home and at school have also been suggested to be a pragmatic and effective way in modifying the profile of risk and protective factors for adolescent suicides (384). It is hoped that future research, ideally involving robust RCTs focusing on adolescents, with larger sample sizes and longer follow-up periods, would support the implementation of an effective mixture of population-based, public health approaches and personalised therapeutic interventions to reduce adolescent self-harm behaviour.

References

1. Favazza AR, Favazza B. Bodies under siege: self-mutilation in culture and psychiatry. Baltimore: MD: Johns Hopkins University Press; 1987.

2. Menninger KA. Man against himself. Oxford, UK: Harcourt, Brace; 1938.

3. Kreitman N, Philip AE, Greer S, Bagley CR. Parasuicide. British Journal of Psychiatry. 1969;115:746-7.

4. Hjelmeland H, Hawton K, Nordvik H, Bille-Brahe U, De Leo D, Fekete S, *et al.* Why people engage in parasuicide: a cross-cultural study of intentions. Suicide Life Threat Behav. 2002;32:380-93.

5. Schmidtke A, Bille-Brahe U, DeLeo D, Kerkhof A, Bjerke T, Crepet P, *et al.* Attempted suicide in Europe: rates, trends and sociodemographic characteristics of suicide attempters during the period 1989-1992. Results of the WHO/EURO Multicentre Study on Parasuicide. Acta Psychiatr Scand. 1996;93:327-38.

6. Beck AT, Beck R, Kovacs M. Classification of suicidal behaviors: I. Quantifying intent and medical lethality. Am J Psychiatry. 1975;132: 285-7.

7. Beck ATe, Lettieri DJe, Resnik HLPe. The Prediction of suicide. Bowie, Md.: Charles Press Publishers; 1974.

8. Merriam-Webster Dictionary [cited 2015 July 20]. Available from: http://www.merriam-webster.com/dictionary/intent

9.   Andriessen K. On "intention" in the definition of suicide. Suicide Life Threat Behav. 2006;36:533-8.

10.   Hawton K, Heeringen Kv. The international handbook of suicide and attempted suicide. Chichester: John Wiley; 2000. xviii, 755 p. p.

11.   Hawton K, Rodham K, Evans E, Weatherall R. Deliberate self harm in adolescents: self report survey in schools in England. BMJ. 2002;325:1207-11.

12.   Freeman D, Wilson K, Thigpen J, McGee R. Assessing intention to die in self-injury behavior. In: Neuringer C, editor. Psychological assessment of suicidal risk. Oxford, UK: Charles C Thomas; 1974.

13.   Pierce DW. Suicidal intent in self-injury. The British journal of psychiatry : the journal of mental science. 1977;130:377-85.

14.   Harriss L, Hawton K. Suicidal intent in deliberate self-harm and the risk of suicide: The predictive power of the Suicide Intent Scale. Journal of Affective Disorders. 2005;86:225-33.

15.   Posner K, Oquendo MA, Gould M, Stanley B, Davies M. Columbia Classification Algorithm of Suicide Assessment (C-CASA): Classification of suicidal events in the FDA's pediatric suicidal risk analysis of antidepressants. American Journal of Psychiatry. 2007;164:1035-43.

16.   Jacobs D. The Harvard Medical School guide to suicide assessment and intervention. San Francisco: Jossey-Bass; 1998.

17.   Maris RW, American Association of Suicidology. Assessment and prediction of suicide. New York: Guilford Press; 1992. xxii, 697 p. p.

18.   Brent DA, Perper JA, Goldstein CE, Kolko DJ, Allan MJ, Allman CJ, et al. Risk factors for adolescent suicide. A comparison of adolescent suicide victims with suicidal inpatients. Arch Gen Psychiatry. 1988;45(6):581-8.

19.   Haw C, Hawton K, Houston K, Townsend E. Correlates of relative lethality and suicidal intent among deliberate self-harm patients. Suicide & life-threatening behavior. 2003;33:353-64.

20.   Douglas J, Cooper J, Amos T, Webb R, Guthrie E, Appleby L. "Near-fatal" deliberate self-harm: characteristics, prevention and implications for the prevention of suicide. J Affect Disord. 2004;79:263-8.

21.   Brown GK, Henriques GR, Sosdjan D, Beck AT. Suicide intent and accurate expectations of lethality: predictors of medical lethality of suicide attempts. J Consult Clin Psychol. 2004;72:1170-4.

22.   Carter GL, Clover K, Whyte IM, Dawson AH, D'Este C. Postcards from the EDge project: randomised controlled trial of an intervention using postcards to reduce repetition of hospital treated deliberate self poisoning. BMJ. 2005;331:805.

23.   Harrington R, Kerfoot M, Dyer E, McNiven F, Gill J, Harrington V, *et al.* Randomized trial of a home-based family intervention for children who have deliberately poisoned themselves. J Am Acad Child Adolesc Psychiatry. 1998;37:512-8.

24.   Hawton K, Harriss L, Simkin S, Bale E, Bond A. Self-cutting: patient characteristics compared with self-poisoners. Suicide Life Threat Behav. 2004;34:199-208.

25.   Silverman MM, Berman AL, Sanddal ND, O'Carroll PW, Joiner TE. Rebuilding the tower of Babel: a revised nomenclature for the study of suicide and suicidal behaviors. Part 1: Background, rationale, and methodology. Suicide Life Threat Behav. 2007;37:248-63.

26.   Hawton K, Harriss L, Hall S, Simkin S, Bale E, Bond A. Deliberate self-harm in Oxford, 1990-2000: a time of change in patient characteristics. Psychol Med. 2003;33:987-95.

27.   De Leo D, Burgis S, Bertolote JM, Kerkhof AJ, Bille-Brahe U. Definitions of suicidal behavior: lessons learned from the WHO/ EURO multicentre Study. Crisis. 2006;27:4-15.

28.   Haw C, Hawton K, Houston K, Townsend E. Psychiatric and personality disorders in deliberate self-harm patients. British Journal of Psychiatry. 2001;178:48-54.

29.   Haw C, Hawton K. Life problems and deliberate self-harm: Associations with gender, age, suicidal intent and psychiatric and personality disorder. Journal of Affective Disorders. 2008;109:139-48.

30.   Crane C, Williams JMG, Hawton K, Arensman E, Hjelmeland H, Bille-Brahe U, *et al.* The association between life events and suicide intent in self-poisoners with and without a history of deliberate self-

harm: a preliminary study. Suicide & life-threatening behavior. 2007;37:367-78.

31. Liang S, Yan J, Zhang T, Zhu C, Situ M, Du N, *et al.* Differences between non-suicidal self injury and suicide attempt in Chinese adolescents. Asian Journal of Psychiatry. 2014;8:76-83.

32. Ougrin D, Zundel T, Kyriakopoulos M, Banarsee R, Stahl D, Taylor E. Adolescents with suicidal and nonsuicidal self-harm: clinical characteristics and response to therapeutic assessment. Psychol Assess. 2012;24(1):11-20.

33. Brausch AM, Gutierrez PM. Differences in non-suicidal self-injury and suicide attempts in adolescents. Journal of Youth and Adolescence. 2010;39:233-42.

34. Butler AM, Malone K. Attempted suicide v. non-suicidal self-injury: Behaviour syndrome or diagnosis? 2013. p. 324-5.

35. Muehlenkamp JJ, Claes L, Havertape L, Plener PL. International prevalence of adolescent non-suicidal self-injury and deliberate self-harm. 2012. p. 10-.

36. Andover MS, Morris BW, Wren A, Bruzzese ME. The co-occurrence of non-suicidal self-injury and attempted suicide among adolescents: distinguishing risk factors and psychosocial correlates. 2012. p. 11-.

37. Wilkinson P, Kelvin R, Roberts C, Dubicka B, Goodyer I. Clinical and psychosocial predictors of suicide attempts and nonsuicidal self-injury in the Adolescent Depression Antidepressants and Psycho-therapy Trial (ADAPT). American Journal of Psychiatry. 2011;168: 495-501.

38. Andover MS, Gibb BE. Non-suicidal self-injury, attempted suicide, and suicidal intent among psychiatric inpatients. Psychiatry Research. 2010;178:101-5.

39. Asarnow JR, Porta G, Spirito A, Emslie G, Clarke G, Wagner KD, *et al.* Suicide attempts and nonsuicidal self-injury in the treatment of resistant depression in adolescents: findings from the TORDIA study. J Am Acad Child Adolesc Psychiatry. 2011;50(8):772-81.

40. Nock MK. Self-injury. Annu Rev Clin Psychol. 2010;6:339-63.

41.   Bergen H, Hawton K, Waters K, Ness J, Cooper J, Steeg S, *et al.* How do methods of non-fatal self-harm relate to eventual suicide? Journal of Affective Disorders. 2012;136:526-33.

42.   American Psychiatric A. Diagnostic and Statistical Manual of Mental Disorders, 5th Edition (DSM-5)2013. 280- p.

43.   Wilkinson P. Non-suicidal self-injury. Eur Child Adolesc Psychiatry. 2013;22 Suppl 1:S75-9.

44.   Nock MK, Prinstein MJ. A functional approach to the assessment of self-mutilative behavior. Journal of consulting and clinical psychology. 2004;72:885-90.

45.   Angold A, Costello EJ. The Child and Adolescent Psychiatric Assessment (CAPA). J Am Acad Child Adolesc Psychiatry. 2000; 39(1):39-48.

46.   Gratz K. Measurement of deliberate self-harm: preliminary data on the deliberate self-harm inventory. Journal of Psychopathology and Behavioral Assessment. 2001;23(4).

47.   Nock MK, Prinstein MJ. A functional approach to the assessment of self-mutilative behavior. J Consult Clin Psychol. 2004;72(5):885-90.

48.   Reich W. Diagnostic interview for children and adolescents (DICA). J Am Acad Child Adolesc Psychiatry. 2000;39(1):59-66.

49.   Gutierrez PM, Osman A, Barrios FX, Kopper BA. Development and initial validation of the Self-harm Behavior Questionnaire. J Pers Assess. 2001;77(3):475-90.

50.   Kaufman J, Birmaher B, Brent D, Rao U, Flynn C, Moreci P, *et al.* Schedule for Affective Disorders and Schizophrenia for School-Age Children-Present and Lifetime Version (K-SADS-PL): initial reliability and validity data. J Am Acad Child Adolesc Psychiatry. 1997; 36(7):980-8.

51.   Ougrin D, Boege I. Brief report: the Self Harm Questionnaire: a new tool designed to improve identification of self harm in adolescents. J Adolesc. 2013;36(1):221-5.

52.   Sansone RA, Wiederman MW, Sansone LA. The Self-Harm Inventory (SHI): development of a scale for identifying self-destructive

behaviors and borderline personality disorder. J Clin Psychol. 1998;54(7):973-83.

53. Tuisku V, Pelkonen M, Karlsson L, Kiviruusu O, Holi M, Ruuttu T, *et al*. Suicidal ideation, deliberate self-harm behaviour and suicide attempts among adolescent outpatients with depressive mood disorders and comorbid axis I disorders. Eur Child Adolesc Psychiatry. 2006;15(4):199-206.

54. Fliege H, Kocalevent RD, Walter OB, Beck S, Gratz KL, Gutierrez PM, *et al*. Three assessment tools for deliberate self-harm and suicide behavior: evaluation and psychopathological correlates. J Psychosom Res. 2006;61(1):113-21.

55. Kapur N, Cooper J, Rodway C, Kelly J, Guthrie E, Mackway-Jones K. Predicting the risk of repetition after self harm: cohort study. BMJ. 2005;330(7488):394-5.

56. Prinstein MJ, Nock MK, Spirito A, Grapentine WL. Multimethod assessment of suicidality in adolescent psychiatric inpatients: preliminary results. J Am Acad Child Adolesc Psychiatry. 2001; 40(9):1053-61.

57. Evans E, Hawton K, Rodham K, Psychol C, Deeks J. The Prevalence of Suicidal Phenomena in Adolescents: A Systematic Review of Population-Based Studies. Suicide and Life-Threatening Behavior. 2005;35:239-50.

58. Mergl R, Koburger N, Heinrichs K, Székely A, Tóth MD, Coyne J, *et al*. What Are Reasons for the Large Gender Differences in the Lethality of Suicidal Acts? An Epidemiological Analysis in Four European Countries. PLoS One. 2015;10(7):e0129062.

59. Madge N, Hewitt A, Hawton K, de Wilde EJ, Corcoran P, Fekete S, *et al*. Deliberate self-harm within an international community sample of young people: comparative findings from the Child & Adolescent Self-harm in Europe (CASE) Study. J Child Psychol Psychiatry. 2008;49:667-77.

60. Madge N, Hawton K, McMahon EM, Corcoran P, De Leo D, de Wilde EJ, *et al*. Psychological characteristics, stressful life events and deliberate self-harm: findings from the Child & Adolescent Self-

harm in Europe (CASE) Study. Eur Child Adolesc Psychiatry. 2011;20(10):499-508.

61.   Wasserman D, Carli V, Wasserman C, Apter A, Balazs J, Bobes J, *et al.* Saving and empowering young lives in Europe (SEYLE): a randomized controlled trial. BMC Public Health. 2010;10:192.

62.   Carli V, Wasserman C, Wasserman D, Sarchiapone M, Apter A, Balazs J, *et al.* The saving and empowering young lives in Europe (SEYLE) randomized controlled trial (RCT): methodological issues and participant characteristics. BMC Public Health. 2013;13:479.

63.   Carli V, Hoven CW, Wasserman C, Chiesa F, Guffanti G, Sarchiapone M, *et al.* A newly identified group of adolescents at "invisible" risk for psychopathology and suicidal behavior: findings from the SEYLE study. World Psychiatry. 2014;13(1):78-86.

64.   Whitlock J, Exner-Cortens D, Purington A. Assessment of nonsuicidal self-injury: development and initial validation of the Non-Suicidal Self-Injury-Assessment Tool (NSSI-AT). Psychol Assess. 2014;26(3):935-46.

65.   Horváth OL, Mészáros G, Balázs J. [Non-suicidal self-injury in adolescents: current issues]. Neuropsychopharmacol Hung. 2015; 17(1):14-22.

66.   Garrison C, Addy C, McKeown R, Cuffe S, Jackson K, Waller J. Nonsuicidal physically self-damaging acts in adolescents. Journal of Child and Family Studies. 1993;2(4):339-52.

67.   Patton GC, Harris R, Carlin JB, Hibbert ME, Coffey C, Schwartz M, *et al.* Adolescent suicidal behaviours: a population-based study of risk. Psychol Med. 1997;27(3):715-24.

68.   Giletta M, Scholte RH, Engels RC, Ciairano S, Prinstein MJ. Adolescent non-suicidal self-injury: a cross-national study of community samples from Italy, the Netherlands and the United States. Psychiatry Res. 2012;197(1-2):66-72.

69.   Baetens I, Claes L, Muehlenkamp J, Grietens H, Onghena P. Non-suicidal and suicidal self-injurious behavior among Flemish adolescents: A web-survey. Arch Suicide Res. 2011;15(1):56-67.

70. Boričević Maršanić V, Aukst Margetić B, Ožanić Bulić S, Đuretić I, Kniewald H, Jukić T, *et al.* Non-suicidal self-injury among psychiatric outpatient adolescent offspring of Croatian posttraumatic stress disorder male war veterans: Prevalence and psychosocial correlates. Int J Soc Psychiatry. 2015;61(3):265-74.

71. Cheung YT, Wong PW, Lee AM, Lam TH, Fan YS, Yip PS. Non-suicidal self-injury and suicidal behavior: prevalence, co-occurrence, and correlates of suicide among adolescents in Hong Kong. Soc Psychiatry Psychiatr Epidemiol. 2013;48(7):1133-44.

72. Garisch JA, Wilson MS. Prevalence, correlates, and prospective predictors of non-suicidal self-injury among New Zealand adolescents: cross-sectional and longitudinal survey data. Child Adolesc Psychiatry Ment Health. 2015;9:28.

73. Bresin K, Schoenleber M. Gender differences in the prevalence of nonsuicidal self-injury: A meta-analysis. Clin Psychol Rev. 2015;38:55-64.

74. Whitlock J, Knox KL. The relationship between self-injurious behavior and suicide in a young adult population. Arch Pediatr Adolesc Med. 2007;161(7):634-40.

75. Yates TM, Tracy AJ, Luthar SS. Nonsuicidal self-injury among "privileged" youths: longitudinal and cross-sectional approaches to developmental process. J Consult Clin Psychol. 2008;76(1):52-62.

76. CDC. WISQARS Nonfatal Injury Reports: Centers for Disease Control and Prevention; 2007 [16 July 2015]. Available from: http://www.cdc.gov/ncipc/wisqars/nonfatal/definitions.htm#self-harm

77. CDC. WISQARS Nonfatal Injury Reports: Centers of Disease Control and Prevention; 2013 [16 July 2015]. Available from: http://webappa.cdc.gov/cgi-bin/broker.exe

78. Hawton K, Casey D, Bale E, Rutherford D, Bergen H, Simkin S, *et al.* Self-Harm in Oxford 2012: University of Oxford; 2012 [16 July 2015]. Available from: http://cebmh.warne.ox.ac.uk/csr/images/annualreport2012.pdf

79.   Hankin BL, Abela JR. Nonsuicidal self-injury in adolescence: pros-
       pective rates and risk factors in a 2½ year longitudinal study.
       Psychiatry Res. 2011;186(1):65-70.

80.   Stallard P, Spears M, Montgomery AA, Phillips R, Sayal K. Self-harm
       in young adolescents (12-16 years): onset and short-term contin-
       uation in a community sample. BMC Psychiatry. 2013;13:328.

81.   Fergusson DM, Horwood LJ, Ridder EM, Beautrais AL. Suicidal
       behaviour in adolescence and subsequent mental health outcomes in
       young adulthood. Psychol Med. 2005;35(7):983-93.

82.   Mars B, Heron J, Crane C, Hawton K, Lewis G, Macleod J, *et al.*
       Clinical and social outcomes of adolescent self harm: population
       based birth cohort study. BMJ. 2014;349:g5954.

83.   Hawton K, Harriss L. Deliberate self-harm in young people: charac-
       teristics and subsequent mortality in a 20-year cohort of patients
       presenting to hospital. J Clin Psychiatry. 2007;68(10):1574-83.

84.   Steinhausen HC, Bösiger R, Metzke CW. Stability, correlates, and
       outcome of adolescent suicidal risk. J Child Psychol Psychiatry.
       2006;47(7):713-22.

85.   Moran P, Coffey C, Romaniuk H, Olsson C, Borschmann R, Carlin
       JB, *et al.* The natural history of self-harm from adolescence to young
       adulthood: a population-based cohort study. Lancet. 2012;
       379(9812):236-43.

86.   Kann L, Kinchen SA, Williams BI, Ross JG, Lowry R, Grunbaum JA,
       et al. Youth risk behavior surveillance--United States, 1999. MMWR
       CDC Surveill Summ. 2000;49(5):1-32.

87.   Kann L, Kinchen S, Shanklin SL, Flint KH, Kawkins J, Harris WA, *et
       al.* Youth risk behavior surveillance--United States, 2013. MMWR
       Surveill Summ. 2014;63 Suppl 4:1-168.

88.   Muehlenkamp JJ, Gutierrez PM. An investigation of differences
       between self-injurious behavior and suicide attempts in a sample of
       adolescents. Suicide Life Threat Behav. 2004;34:12-23.

89.   Muehlenkamp JJ, Gutierrez PM. Risk for suicide attempts among adolescents who engage in non-suicidal self-injury. Arch Suicide Res. 2007;11:69-82.

90.   Gratz KL. Risk factors for deliberate self-harm among female college students: the role and interaction of childhood maltreatment, emotional inexpressivity, and affect intensity/reactivity. The American journal of orthopsychiatry. 2006;76:238-50.

91.   Gratz KL, Conrad SD, Roemer L. Risk factors for deliberate self-harm among college students. The American journal of orthopsychiatry. 2002;72:128-40.

92.   Lahti A, Harju A, Hakko H, Riala K, Räsänen P. Suicide in children and young adolescents: a 25-year database on suicides from Northern Finland. J Psychiatr Res. 2014;58:123-8.

93.   Freuchen A, Kjelsberg E, Lundervold AJ, Grøholt B. Differences between children and adolescents who commit suicide and their peers: A psychological autopsy of suicide victims compared to accident victims and a community sample. Child Adolesc Psychiatry Ment Health. 2012;6:1.

94.   Freuchen A, Kjelsberg E, Lundervold AJ, Grøholt B. Correction: Differences between children and adolescents who commit suicide and their peers: A psychological autopsy of suicide victims compared to accident victims and a community sample. Child Adolesc Psychiatry Ment Health. 2013;7(1):18.

95.   Organisation WH. Preventing Suicide: A Global Imperative. Geneva: World Health Organization; 2014.

96.   Slobodskaya HR, Semenova NB. Child and adolescent mental health problems in Tyva Republic, Russia, as possible risk factors for a high suicide rate. Eur Child Adolesc Psychiatry. 2015.

97.   Ajdacic-Gross V, Weiss MG, Ring M, Hepp U, Bopp M, Gutzwiller F, *et al*. Methods of suicide: international suicide patterns derived from the WHO mortality database. Bull World Health Organ. 2008; 86(9):726-32.

98.   Choi KH, Kim DH. Trend of Suicide Rates According to Urbanity among Adolescents by Gender and Suicide Method in Korea, 1997-2012. Int J Environ Res Public Health. 2015;12(5):5129-42.

99.   Hepp U, Stulz N, Unger-Köppel J, Ajdacic-Gross V. Methods of suicide used by children and adolescents. Eur Child Adolesc Psychiatry. 2012;21(2):67-73.

100. Favazza AR. Bodies under siege : self-mutilation, nonsuicidal self-injury, and body modification in culture and psychiatry. 3rd ed. Baltimore: Johns Hopkins University Press; 2011. xv, 333 p. p.

101. Brent D. What family studies teach us about suicidal behavior: implications for research, treatment, and prevention. Eur Psychiatry. 2010;25(5):260-3.

102. Brent DA, Bridge J, Johnson BA, Connolly J. Suicidal behavior runs in families. A controlled family study of adolescent suicide victims. Arch Gen Psychiatry. 1996;53(12):1145-52.

103. Mittendorfer-Rutz E, Rasmussen F, Wasserman D. Familial clustering of suicidal behaviour and psychopathology in young suicide attempters. A register-based nested case control study. Soc Psychiatry Psychiatr Epidemiol. 2008;43(1):28-36.

104. Brent DA, Oquendo M, Birmaher B, Greenhill L, Kolko D, Stanley B, et al. Peripubertal suicide attempts in offspring of suicide attempters with siblings concordant for suicidal behavior. Am J Psychiatry. 2003;160(8):1486-93.

105. Geulayov G, Gunnell D, Holmen TL, Metcalfe C. The association of parental fatal and non-fatal suicidal behaviour with offspring suicidal behaviour and depression: a systematic review and meta-analysis. Psychol Med. 2012;42(8):1567-80.

106. Voracek M, Loibl LM. Genetics of suicide: A systematic review of twin studies. Wiener Klinische Wochenschrift. 2007;119(15-16):463-75.

107. Segal NL. Suicidal behaviors in surviving monozygotic and dizygotic co-twins: is the nature of the co-twin's cause of death a factor? Suicide Life Threat Behav. 2009;39(6):569-75.

108. Lieb R, Bronisch T, Höfler M, Schreier A, Wittchen HU. Maternal suicidality and risk of suicidality in offspring: findings from a community study. Am J Psychiatry. 2005;162(9):1665-71.

109. Maciejewski DF, Creemers HE, Lynskey MT, Madden PA, Heath AC, Statham DJ, *et al.* Overlapping genetic and environmental influences on nonsuicidal self-injury and suicidal ideation: different outcomes, same etiology? JAMA Psychiatry. 2014;71(6):699-705.

110. Kim-Cohen J, Caspi A, Taylor A, Williams B, Newcombe R, Craig IW, *et al.* MAOA, maltreatment, and gene-environment interaction predicting children's mental health: new evidence and a meta-analysis. Mol Psychiatry. 2006;11(10):903-13.

111. Slap G, Goodman E, Huang B. Adoption as a risk factor for attempted suicide during adolescence. Pediatrics. 2001;108(2):E30.

112. Voracek M. Genetic factors in suicide: reassessment of adoption studies and individuals' beliefs about adoption study findings. Psychiatr Danub. 2007;19(3):139-53.

113. Petersen L, Sørensen TI, Kragh Andersen P, Mortensen PB, Hawton K. Genetic and familial environmental effects on suicide attempts: a study of Danish adoptees and their biological and adoptive siblings. J Affect Disord. 2014;155:273-7.

114. Petersen L, Sørensen TI, Andersen PK, Mortensen PB, Hawton K. Genetic and familial environmental effects on suicide--an adoption study of siblings. PLoS One. 2013;8(10):e77973.

115. von Borczyskowski A, Lindblad F, Vinnerljung B, Reintjes R, Hjern A. Familial factors and suicide: an adoption study in a Swedish National Cohort. Psychol Med. 2011;41(4):749-58.

116. Jorgensen TJ, Ruczinski I, Kessing B, Smith MW, Shugart YY, Alberg AJ. Hypothesis-driven candidate gene association studies: practical design and analytical considerations. Am J Epidemiol. 2009;170(8):986-93.

117. Terwilliger JD, Göring HH. Gene mapping in the 20th and 21st centuries: statistical methods, data analysis, and experimental design. Hum Biol. 2000;72(1):63-132.

118. Gottesman II, Gould TD. The endophenotype concept in psychiatry: etymology and strategic intentions. Am J Psychiatry. 2003;160(4):636-45.

119. Mann JJ, Arango VA, Avenevoli S, Brent DA, Champagne FA, Clayton P, *et al.* Candidate endophenotypes for genetic studies of suicidal behavior. Biol Psychiatry. 2009;65(7):556-63.

120. Evans J, Platts H, Liebenau A. Impulsiveness and deliberate self-harm: a comparison of "first-timers' and "repeaters'. Acta Psychiatr Scand. 1996;93(5):378-80.

121. Kirby LG, Zeeb FD, Winstanley CA. Contributions of serotonin in addiction vulnerability. Neuropharmacology. 2011;61(3):421-32.

122. Winstanley CA, Theobald DE, Dalley JW, Robbins TW. Interactions between serotonin and dopamine in the control of impulsive choice in rats: therapeutic implications for impulse control disorders. Neuropsychopharmacology. 2005;30(4):669-82.

123. Young SN, Leyton M. The role of serotonin in human mood and social interaction. Insight from altered tryptophan levels. Pharmacol Biochem Behav. 2002;71(4):857-65.

124. Mann JJ, Brent DA, Arango V. The neurobiology and genetics of suicide and attempted suicide: A focus on the serotonergic system. 2001. p. 467-77.

125. Antypa N, Serretti A, Rujescu D. Serotonergic genes and suicide: a systematic review. Eur Neuropsychopharmacol. 2013;23(10):1125-42.

126. Bellivier F, Chaste P, Malafosse A. Association between the TPH gene A218C polymorphism and suicidal behavior: a meta-analysis. Am J Med Genet B Neuropsychiatr Genet. 2004;124B(1):87-91.

127. Li D, He L. Further clarification of the contribution of the tryptophan hydroxylase (TPH) gene to suicidal behavior using systematic allelic and genotypic meta-analyses. Hum Genet. 2006;119(3):233-40.

128. González-Castro TB, Juárez-Rojop I, López-Narváez ML, Tovilla-Zárate CA. Association of TPH-1 and TPH-2 gene polymorphisms with suicidal behavior: a systematic review and meta-analysis. BMC Psychiatry. 2014;14:196.

129. de Medeiros Alves V, Bezerra DG, de Andrade TG, de Melo Neto VL, Nardi AE. Genetic Polymorphisms Might Predict Suicide Attempts in Mental Disorder Patients: A Systematic Review And Meta-Analysis. CNS Neurol Disord Drug Targets. 2015;14(7):820-7.

130. Oquendo MA, Mann JJ. The biology of impulsivity and suicidality. Psychiatr Clin North Am. 2000;23(1):11-25.

131. Pandey GN, Dwivedi Y. Noradrenergic function in suicide. Arch Suicide Res. 2007;11(3):235-46.

132. Daubner SC, Le T, Wang S. Tyrosine hydroxylase and regulation of dopamine synthesis. Arch Biochem Biophys. 2011;508(1):1-12.

133. Giegling I, Moreno-De-Luca D, Rujescu D, Schneider B, Hartmann AM, Schnabel A, et al. Dopa decarboxylase and tyrosine hydroxylase gene variants in suicidal behavior. Am J Med Genet B Neuropsychiatr Genet. 2008;147(3):308-15.

134. Fukutake M, Hishimoto A, Nishiguchi N, Nushida H, Ueno Y, Shirakawa O, et al. Association of alpha2A-adrenergic receptor gene polymorphism with susceptibility to suicide in Japanese females. Prog Neuropsychopharmacol Biol Psychiatry. 2008;32(6):1428-33.

135. Hosák L. Role of the COMT gene Val158Met polymorphism in mental disorders: a review. Eur Psychiatry. 2007;22(5):276-81.

136. Kia-Keating BM, Glatt SJ, Tsuang MT. Meta-analyses suggest association between COMT, but not HTR1B, alleles, and suicidal behavior. Am J Med Genet B Neuropsychiatr Genet. 2007;144B(8):1048-53.

137. Calati R, Porcelli S, Giegling I, Hartmann AM, Möller HJ, De Ronchi D, et al. Catechol-o-methyltransferase gene modulation on suicidal behavior and personality traits: review, meta-analysis and association study. J Psychiatr Res. 2011;45(3):309-21.

138. Tovilla-Zárate C, Juárez-Rojop I, Ramón-Frias T, Villar-Soto M, Pool-García S, Medellín BC, et al. No association between COMT val158met polymorphism and suicidal behavior: meta-analysis and new data. BMC Psychiatry. 2011;11:151.

139. Cheng WW, Jia CX, Pan YF, Zhao SY, Jia GY, Hu MH. [The relationship between gene polymorphism of catechol-O-methyltransferase and survival of oral pesticides suicide attempters]. Zhonghua Nei Ke Za Zhi. 2006;45(5):403-5.

140. Baud P, Courtet P, Perroud N, Jollant F, Buresi C, Malafosse A. Catechol-O-methyltransferase polymorphism (COMT) in suicide attempters: a possible gender effect on anger traits. Am J Med Genet B Neuropsychiatr Genet. 2007;144B(8):1042-7.

141. Lee LO, Prescott CA. Association of the catechol-O-methyltransferase val158met polymorphism and anxiety-related traits: a meta-analysis. Psychiatr Genet. 2014;24(2):52-69.

142. Nedic G, Nikolac M, Sviglin KN, Muck-Seler D, Borovecki F, Pivac N. Association study of a functional catechol-O-methyltransferase (COMT) Val108/158Met polymorphism and suicide attempts in patients with alcohol dependence. Int J Neuropsychopharmacol. 2011;14(3):377-88.

143. Persson ML, Geijer T, Wasserman D, Rockah R, Frisch A, Michaelovsky E, et al. Lack of association between suicide attempt and a polymorphism at the dopamine receptor D4 locus. Psychiatr Genet. 1999;9(2):97-100.

144. Zalsman G, Frisch A, Lewis R, Michaelovsky E, Hermesh H, Sher L, et al. DRD4 receptor gene exon III polymorphism in inpatient suicidal adolescents. J Neural Transm. 2004;111(12):1593-603.

145. Munafò MR, Yalcin B, Willis-Owen SA, Flint J. Association of the dopamine D4 receptor (DRD4) gene and approach-related personality traits: meta-analysis and new data. Biol Psychiatry. 2008; 63(2):197-206.

146. Barzman D, Geise C, Lin PI. Review of the genetic basis of emotion dysregulation in children and adolescents. World J Psychiatry. 2015;5(1):112-7.

147. Skaper SD. The neurotrophin family of neurotrophic factors: an overview. Methods Mol Biol. 2012;846:1-12.

148. Yoshimura R, Ikenouchi-Sugita A, Hori H, Umene-Nakano W, Katsuki A, Hayashi K, et al. [Brain-derived neurotrophic factor

(BDNF) and mood disorder]. Nihon Shinkei Seishin Yakurigaku Zasshi. 2010;30(5-6):181-4.

149. Pandey GN, Ren X, Rizavi HS, Conley RR, Roberts RC, Dwivedi Y. Brain-derived neurotrophic factor and tyrosine kinase B receptor signalling in post-mortem brain of teenage suicide victims. Int J Neuropsychopharmacol. 2008;11(8):1047-61.

150. Banerjee R, Ghosh AK, Ghosh B, Bhattacharyya S, Mondal AC. Decreased mRNA and Protein Expression of BDNF, NGF, and their Receptors in the Hippocampus from Suicide: An Analysis in Human Postmortem Brain. Clin Med Insights Pathol. 2013;6:1-11.

151. Dwivedi Y. The neurobiological basis of suicide. Boca Raton, FL: Taylor & Francis/CRC Press; 2012.

152. Keller S, Sarchiapone M, Zarrilli F, Videtic A, Ferraro A, Carli V, *et al*. Increased BDNF promoter methylation in the Wernicke area of suicide subjects. Arch Gen Psychiatry. 2010;67(3):258-67.

153. Keller S, Sarchiapone M, Zarrilli F, Tomaiuolo R, Carli V, Angrisano T, *et al*. TrkB gene expression and DNA methylation state in Wernicke area does not associate with suicidal behavior. J Affect Disord. 2011;135(1-3):400-4.

154. Kang HJ, Kim JM, Lee JY, Kim SY, Bae KY, Kim SW, *et al*. BDNF promoter methylation and suicidal behavior in depressive patients. J Affect Disord. 2013;151(2):679-85.

155. Kim JM, Kang HJ, Bae KY, Kim SW, Shin IS, Kim HR, *et al*. Association of BDNF promoter methylation and genotype with suicidal ideation in elderly Koreans. Am J Geriatr Psychiatry. 2014;22(10):989-96.

156. Kim JM, Kang HJ, Kim SY, Kim SW, Shin IS, Kim HR, *et al*. BDNF promoter methylation associated with suicidal ideation in patients with breast cancer. Int J Psychiatry Med. 2015;49(1):75-94.

157. Jiang X, Xu K, Hoberman J, Tian F, Marko AJ, Waheed JF, *et al*. BDNF variation and mood disorders: a novel functional promoter polymorphism and Val66Met are associated with anxiety but have opposing effects. Neuropsychopharmacology. 2005;30(7):1353-61.

158. Gatt JM, Nemeroff CB, Dobson-Stone C, Paul RH, Bryant RA, Schofield PR, *et al.* Interactions between BDNF Val66Met polymorphism and early life stress predict brain and arousal pathways to syndromal depression and anxiety. Mol Psychiatry. 2009;14(7):681-95.

159. Groves JO. Is it time to reassess the BDNF hypothesis of depression? Mol Psychiatry. 2007;12(12):1079-88.

160. Kim B, Kim CY, Hong JP, Kim SY, Lee C, Joo YH. Brain-derived neurotrophic factor Val/Met polymorphism and bipolar disorder. Association of the Met allele with suicidal behavior of bipolar patients. Neuropsychobiology. 2008;58(2):97-103.

161. Sarchiapone M, Carli V, Roy A, Iacoviello L, Cuomo C, Latella MC, *et al.* Association of polymorphism (Val66Met) of brain-derived neurotrophic factor with suicide attempts in depressed patients. Neuropsychobiology. 2008;57(3):139-45.

162. Schenkel LC, Segal J, Becker JA, Manfro GG, Bianchin MM, Leistner-Segal S. The BDNF Val66Met polymorphism is an independent risk factor for high lethality in suicide attempts of depressed patients. Prog Neuropsychopharmacol Biol Psychiatry. 2010;34(6):940-4.

163. Zarrilli F, Angiolillo A, Castaldo G, Chiariotti L, Keller S, Sacchetti S, *et al.* Brain derived neurotrophic factor (BDNF) genetic polymorphism (Val66Met) in suicide: a study of 512 cases. Am J Med Genet B Neuropsychiatr Genet. 2009;150B(4):599-600.

164. Wang C, Zhang Y, Liu B, Long H, Yu C, Jiang T. Dosage effects of BDNF Val66Met polymorphism on cortical surface area and functional connectivity. J Neurosci. 2014;34(7):2645-51.

165. Beevers CG, Wells TT, McGeary JE. The BDNF Val66Met polymorphism is associated with rumination in healthy adults. Emotion. 2009;9(4):579-84.

166. Ambrus L, Träskman-Bendz L, Westrin Å, Sunnqvist C, Ekman A, Suchankova P. Associations between avoidant focused coping strategies and polymorphisms in genes coding for brain-derived neurotrophic factor and vascular endothelial growth factor in suicide attempters: a preliminary study. Psychiatry Res. 2014;220(1-2):732-3.

167. Zai CC, Manchia M, De Luca V, Tiwari AK, Chowdhury NI, Zai GC, *et al.* The brain-derived neurotrophic factor gene in suicidal behaviour: a meta-analysis. Int J Neuropsychopharmacol. 2012; 15(8):1037-42.

168. Paska AV, Zupanc T, Pregelj P. The role of brain-derived neurotrophic factor in the pathophysiology of suicidal behavior. Psychiatr Danub. 2013;25 Suppl 2:S341-4.

169. Perroud N, Courtet P, Vincze I, Jaussent I, Jollant F, Bellivier F, *et al.* Interaction between BDNF Val66Met and childhood trauma on adult's violent suicide attempt. Genes Brain Behav. 2008;7(3):314-22.

170. Pregelj P, Nedic G, Paska AV, Zupanc T, Nikolac M, Balažic J, *et al.* The association between brain-derived neurotrophic factor polymorphism (BDNF Val66Met) and suicide. J Affect Disord. 2011; 128(3):287-90.

171. Sher L. The role of brain-derived neurotrophic factor in the pathophysiology of adolescent suicidal behavior. Int J Adolesc Med Health. 2011;23(3):181-5.

172. Bresin K, Sima Finy M, Verona E. Childhood emotional environment and self-injurious behaviors: the moderating role of the BDNF Val66Met polymorphism. J Affect Disord. 2013;150(2):594-600.

173. Lockwood LE, Su S, Youssef NA. The role of epigenetics in depression and suicide: A platform for gene-environment interactions. Psychiatry Res. 2015.

174. Schneider E, El Hajj N, Müller F, Navarro B, Haaf T. Epigenetic Dysregulation in the Prefrontal Cortex of Suicide Completers. Cytogenet Genome Res. 2015.

175. Stanley M, Mann JJ. Increased serotonin-2 binding sites in frontal cortex of suicide victims. Lancet. 1983;1(8318):214-6.

176. Asberg M. Neurotransmitters and suicidal behavior. The evidence from cerebrospinal fluid studies. Ann N Y Acad Sci. 1997;836:158-81.

177. van Praag HM. CSF 5-HIAA and suicide in non-depressed schizophrenics. Lancet. 1983;2(8356):977-8.

178. Jokinen J, Nordström AL, Nordström P. CSF 5-HIAA and DST non-suppression--orthogonal biologic risk factors for suicide in male mood disorder inpatients. Psychiatry Res. 2009;165(1-2):96-102.

179. Nordström P, Samuelsson M, Asberg M, Träskman-Bendz L, Aberg-Wistedt A, Nordin C, *et al.* CSF 5-HIAA predicts suicide risk after attempted suicide. Suicide Life Threat Behav. 1994;24(1):1-9.

180. Chatzittofis A, Nordström P, Hellström C, Arver S, Åsberg M, Jokinen J. CSF 5-HIAA, cortisol and DHEAS levels in suicide attempters. Eur Neuropsychopharmacol. 2013;23(10):1280-7.

181. Samuelsson M, Jokinen J, Nordström AL, Nordström P. CSF 5-HIAA, suicide intent and hopelessness in the prediction of early suicide in male high-risk suicide attempters. Acta Psychiatr Scand. 2006;113(1):44-7.

182. Mehlman PT, Higley JD, Faucher I, Lilly AA, Taub DM, Vickers J, *et al.* Low CSF 5-HIAA concentrations and severe aggression and impaired impulse control in nonhuman primates. Am J Psychiatry. 1994;151(10):1485-91.

183. Cremniter D, Jamain S, Kollenbach K, Alvarez JC, Lecrubier Y, Gilton A, *et al.* CSF 5-HIAA levels are lower in impulsive as compared to nonimpulsive violent suicide attempters and control subjects. Biol Psychiatry. 1999;45(12):1572-9.

184. Pandey GN, Dwivedi Y, Rizavi HS, Ren X, Pandey SC, Pesold C, *et al.* Higher expression of serotonin 5-HT(2A) receptors in the postmortem brains of teenage suicide victims. Am J Psychiatry. 2002;159(3):419-29.

185. Boulougouris V, Malogiannis I, Lockwood G, Zervas I, Di Giovanni G. Serotonergic modulation of suicidal behaviour: integrating preclinical data with clinical practice and psychotherapy. Exp Brain Res. 2013;230(4):605-24.

186. van Heeringen C, Audenaert K, Van Laere K, Dumont F, Slegers G, Mertens J, *et al.* Prefrontal 5-HT2a receptor binding index, hopelessness and personality characteristics in attempted suicide. J Affect Disord. 2003;74(2):149-58.

187. Oquendo MA, Russo SA, Underwood MD, Kassir SA, Ellis SP, Mann JJ, *et al.* Higher postmortem prefrontal 5-HT2A receptor binding correlates with lifetime aggression in suicide. Biol Psychiatry. 2006;59(3):235-43.

188. Audenaert K, Van Laere K, Dumont F, Slegers G, Mertens J, van Heeringen C, *et al.* Decreased frontal serotonin 5-HT 2a receptor binding index in deliberate self-harm patients. Eur J Nucl Med. 2001;28(2):175-82.

189. Lauterbach E, Brunner J, Hawellek B, Lewitzka U, Ising M, Bondy B, *et al.* Platelet 5-HT2A receptor binding and tryptophan availability in depression are not associated with recent history of suicide attempts but with personality traits characteristic for suicidal behavior. J Affect Disord. 2006;91(1):57-62.

190. Roggenbach J, Müller-Oerlinghausen B, Franke L, Uebelhack R, Blank S, Ahrens B. Peripheral serotonergic markers in acutely suicidal patients. 1. Comparison of serotonergic platelet measures between suicidal individuals, nonsuicidal patients with major depression and healthy subjects. J Neural Transm. 2007;114(4):479-87.

191. Pandey GN. Signal transduction abnormalities in suicide: focus on phosphoinositide signaling system. CNS Neurol Disord Drug Targets. 2013;12(7):941-53.

192. Purselle DC, Nemeroff CB. Serotonin transporter: a potential substrate in the biology of suicide. Neuropsychopharmacology. 2003;28(4):613-9.

193. Mann JJ, Huang YY, Underwood MD, Kassir SA, Oppenheim S, Kelly TM, *et al.* A serotonin transporter gene promoter poly-morphism (5-HTTLPR) and prefrontal cortical binding in major depression and suicide. Arch Gen Psychiatry. 2000;57(8):729-38.

194. Matsumoto R, Ichise M, Ito H, Ando T, Takahashi H, Ikoma Y, *et al.* Reduced serotonin transporter binding in the insular cortex in patients with obsessive-compulsive disorder: a [11C]DASB PET study. Neuroimage. 2010;49(1):121-6.

195. McCann UD, Szabo Z, Seckin E, Rosenblatt P, Mathews WB, Ravert HT, *et al.* Quantitative PET studies of the serotonin transporter in MDMA users and controls using [11C]McN5652 and [11C]DASB. Neuropsychopharmacology. 2005;30(9):1741-50.

196. Picouto MD, Villar F, Braquehais MD. The role of serotonin in adolescent suicide: theoretical, methodological, and clinical concerns. Int J Adolesc Med Health. 2015;27(2):129-33.

197. Groschwitz RC, Plener PL. The Neurobiology of Non-Suicidal Self-Injury (NSSI): A review. Suicidology Online. 2012;3:24-32.

198. Crowell SE, Beauchaine TP, McCauley E, Smith CJ, Vasilev CA, Stevens AL. Parent-child interactions, peripheral serotonin, and self-inflicted injury in adolescents. J Consult Clin Psychol. 2008;76(1):15-21.

199. Mann JJ, Brent DA, Arango V. The neurobiology and genetics of suicide and attempted suicide: a focus on the serotonergic system. Neuropsychopharmacology. 2001;24(5):467-77.

200. Pariante CM, Lightman SL. The HPA axis in major depression: classical theories and new developments. Trends Neurosci. 2008;31(9):464-8.

201. Daban C, Vieta E, Mackin P, Young AH. Hypothalamic-pituitary-adrenal axis and bipolar disorder. Psychiatr Clin North Am. 2005;28(2):469-80.

202. Young EA, Abelson JL, Cameron OG. Interaction of brain noradrenergic system and the hypothalamic-pituitary-adrenal (HPA) axis in man. Psychoneuroendocrinology. 2005;30(8):807-14.

203. Oquendo MA, Sullivan GM, Sudol K, Baca-Garcia E, Stanley BH, Sublette ME, *et al.* Toward a biosignature for suicide. Am J Psychiatry. 2014;171(12):1259-77.

204. Pfeffer CR, Stokes P, Shindledecker R. Suicidal behavior and hypothalamic-pituitary-adrenocortical axis indices in child psychiatric inpatients. Biol Psychiatry. 1991;29(9):909-17.

205. Dahl RE, Kaufman J, Ryan ND, Perel J, al-Shabbout M, Birmaher B, *et al.* The dexamethasone suppression test in children and

adolescents: a review and a controlled study. Biol Psychiatry. 1992;32(2):109-26.

206. Kaess M, Hille M, Parzer P, Maser-Gluth C, Resch F, Brunner R. Alterations in the neuroendocrinological stress response to acute psychosocial stress in adolescents engaging in nonsuicidal self-injury. Psychoneuroendocrinology. 2012;37(1):157-61.

207. Beauchaine TP, Crowell SE, Hsiao RC. Post-dexamethasone cortisol, self-inflicted injury, and suicidal ideation among depressed adolescent girls. J Abnorm Child Psychol. 2015;43(4):619-32.

208. Coryell W, Schlesser M. The dexamethasone suppression test and suicide prediction. Am J Psychiatry. 2001;158(5):748-53.

209. Westrin A, Niméus A. The dexamethasone suppression test and CSF-5-HIAA in relation to suicidality and depression in suicide attempters. Eur Psychiatry. 2003;18(4):166-71.

210. Jokinen J, Mårtensson B, Nordström AL, Nordström P. CSF 5-HIAA and DST non-suppression -independent biomarkers in suicide attempters? J Affect Disord. 2008;105(1-3):241-5.

211. Sher L. The role of the hypothalamic-pituitary-adrenal axis dysfunction in the pathophysiology of alcohol misuse and suicidal behavior in adolescents. Int J Adolesc Med Health. 2007;19(1):3-9.

212. Jokinen J, Nordström P. HPA axis hyperactivity as suicide predictor in elderly mood disorder inpatients. Psychoneuroendocrinology. 2008;33(10):1387-93.

213. Jokinen J, Nordström P. HPA axis hyperactivity and attempted suicide in young adult mood disorder inpatients. J Affect Disord. 2009;116(1-2):117-20.

214. Kamali M, Saunders EF, Prossin AR, Brucksch CB, Harrington GJ, Langenecker SA, *et al.* Associations between suicide attempts and elevated bedtime salivary cortisol levels in bipolar disorder. J Affect Disord. 2012;136(3):350-8.

215. Braquehais MD, Picouto MD, Casas M, Sher L. Hypothalamic-pituitary-adrenal axis dysfunction as a neurobiological correlate of

emotion dysregulation in adolescent suicide. World J Pediatr. 2012;8(3):197-206.

216. Lindqvist D, Isaksson A, Träskman-Bendz L, Brundin L. Salivary cortisol and suicidal behavior--a follow-up study. Psychoneuro-endocrinology. 2008;33(8):1061-8.

217. Pompili M, Serafini G, Innamorati M, Möller-Leimkühler AM, Giupponi G, Girardi P, *et al*. The hypothalamic-pituitary-adrenal axis and serotonin abnormalities: a selective overview for the implications of suicide prevention. Eur Arch Psychiatry Clin Neurosci. 2010;260(8):583-600.

218. Watson S, Mackin P. HPA axis function in mood disorders. Psychiatry. 2006;5(5):166-70.

219. Arango V, Underwood MD, Mann JJ. Fewer pigmented locus coeruleus neurons in suicide victims: preliminary results. Biol Psychiatry. 1996;39(2):112-20.

220. Ordway GA. Pathophysiology of the locus coeruleus in suicide. Ann N Y Acad Sci. 1997;836:233-52.

221. Zhu MY, Klimek V, Dilley GE, Haycock JW, Stockmeier C, Overholser JC, *et al*. Elevated levels of tyrosine hydroxylase in the locus coeruleus in major depression. Biol Psychiatry. 1999;46(9):1275-86.

222. Gos T, Krell D, Bielau H, Brisch R, Trübner K, Steiner J, *et al*. Tyrosine hydroxylase immunoreactivity in the locus coeruleus is elevated in violent suicidal depressive patients. Eur Arch Psychiatry Clin Neurosci. 2008;258(8):513-20.

223. Baumann B, Danos P, Diekmann S, Krell D, Bielau H, Geretsegger C, *et al*. Tyrosine hydroxylase immunoreactivity in the locus coeruleus is reduced in depressed non-suicidal patients but normal in depressed suicide patients. Eur Arch Psychiatry Clin Neurosci. 1999;249(4):212-9.

224. Klimek V, Stockmeier C, Overholser J, Meltzer HY, Kalka S, Dilley G, *et al*. Reduced levels of norepinephrine transporters in the locus coeruleus in major depression. J Neurosci. 1997;17(21):8451-8.

225. Hébert C, Habimana A, Elie R, Reader TA. Effects of chronic antidepressant treatments on 5-HT and NA transporters in rat brain: an autoradiographic study. Neurochem Int. 2001;38(1):63-74.

226. Galfalvy H, Currier D, Oquendo MA, Sullivan G, Huang YY, John Mann J. Lower CSF MHPG predicts short-term risk for suicide attempt. Int J Neuropsychopharmacol. 2009;12(10):1327-35.

227. Sher L, Carballo JJ, Grunebaum MF, Burke AK, Zalsman G, Huang YY, et al. A prospective study of the association of cerebrospinal fluid monoamine metabolite levels with lethality of suicide attempts in patients with bipolar disorder. Bipolar Disord. 2006;8(5 Pt 2):543-50.

228. Lindqvist D, Janelidze S, Erhardt S, Träskman-Bendz L, Engström G, Brundin L. CSF biomarkers in suicide attempters--a principal component analysis. Acta Psychiatr Scand. 2011;124(1):52-61.

229. Curzon G. CSF homovanillic acid: an index of dopaminergic activity. Adv Neurol. 1975;9:349-57.

230. Stanley B, Sher L, Wilson S, Ekman R, Huang Yy, Mann JJ. Non-suicidal self-injurious behavior, endogenous opioids and monoamine neurotransmitters. J Affect Disord. 2010;124(1-2):134-40.

231. Engström G, Alling C, Blennow K, Regnéll G, Träskman-Bendz L. Reduced cerebrospinal HVA concentrations and HVA/5-HIAA ratios in suicide attempters. Monoamine metabolites in 120 suicide attempters and 47 controls. Eur Neuropsychopharmacol. 1999;9(5): 399-405.

232. Träskman L, Asberg M, Bertilsson L, Sjöstrand L. Monoamine metabolites in CSF and suicidal behavior. Arch Gen Psychiatry. 1981; 38(6):631-6.

233. Roy A, Agren H, Pickar D, Linnoila M, Doran AR, Cutler NR, et al. Reduced CSF concentrations of homovanillic acid and homovanillic acid to 5-hydroxyindoleacetic acid ratios in depressed patients: relationship to suicidal behavior and dexamethasone nonsuppression. Am J Psychiatry. 1986;143(12):1539-45.

234. Jones JS, Stanley B, Mann JJ, Frances AJ, Guido JR, Traskman-Bendz L, *et al*. CSF 5-HIAA and HVA concentrations in elderly depressed patients who attempted suicide. Am J Psychiatry. 1990;147(9):1225-7.

235. Roy A, Ninan P, Mazonson A, Pickar D, Van Kammen D, Linnoila M, *et al*. CSF monoamine metabolites in chronic schizophrenic patients who attempt suicide. Psychol Med. 1985;15(2):335-40.

236. Jokinen J, Nordström AL, Nordström P. The relationship between CSF HVA/5-HIAA ratio and suicide intent in suicide attempters. Arch Suicide Res. 2007;11(2):187-92.

237. Jokinen J, Nordström AL, Nordström P. Cerebrospinal fluid monoamine metabolites and suicide. Nord J Psychiatry. 2009; 63(4):276-9.

238. Placidi GP, Oquendo MA, Malone KM, Huang YY, Ellis SP, Mann JJ. Aggressivity, suicide attempts, and depression: relationship to cerebrospinal fluid monoamine metabolite levels. Biol Psychiatry. 2001;50(10):783-91.

239. Pitchot W, Reggers J, Pinto E, Hansenne M, Fuchs S, Pirard S, *et al*. Reduced dopaminergic activity in depressed suicides. Psychoneuroendocrinology. 2001;26(3):331-5.

240. Pitchot W, Hansenne M, Gonzalez Moreno A, Pinto E, Reggers J, Fuchs S, *et al*. Reduced dopamine function in depressed patients is related to suicidal behavior but not its lethality. Psychoneuro-endocrinology. 2001;26(7):689-96.

241. Pitchot W, Hansenne M, Ansseau M. Role of dopamine in non-depressed patients with a history of suicide attempts. Eur Psychiatry. 2001;16(7):424-7.

242. Holden JE, Jeong Y, Forrest JM. The endogenous opioid system and clinical pain management. AACN Clin Issues. 2005;16(3):291-301.

243. Kapitzke D, Vetter I, Cabot PJ. Endogenous opioid analgesia in peripheral tissues and the clinical implications for pain control. Ther Clin Risk Manag. 2005;1(4):279-97.

244. Bresin K, Gordon KH. Endogenous opioids and nonsuicidal self-injury: a mechanism of affect regulation. Neurosci Biobehav Rev. 2013;37(3):374-83.

245. Victor SE, Glenn CR, Klonsky ED. Is non-suicidal self-injury an "addiction"? A comparison of craving in substance use and non-suicidal self-injury. Psychiatry Res. 2012;197(1-2):73-7.

246. Sher L, Stanley BH. The role of endogenous opioids in the pathophysiology of self-injurious and suicidal behavior. Arch Suicide Res. 2008;12(4):299-308.

247. Urban MO, Gebhart GF. Central mechanisms in pain. Med Clin North Am. 1999;83(3):585-96.

248. Kuner R. Central mechanisms of pathological pain. Nat Med. 2010;16(11):1258-66.

249. Orbach I, Stein D, Palgi Y, Asherov J, Har-Even D, Elizur A. Perception of physical pain in accident and suicide attempt patients: self-preservation vs self-destruction. J Psychiatr Res. 1996;30(4):307-20.

250. Orbach I, Mikulincer M, King R, Cohen D, Stein D. Thresholds and tolerance of physical pain in suicidal and nonsuicidal adolescents. J Consult Clin Psychol. 1997;65(4):646-52.

251. McCoy K, Fremouw W, McNeil DW. Thresholds and tolerance of physical pain among young adults who self-injure. Pain Res Manag. 2010;15(6):371-7.

252. Hooley JM, Ho DT, Slater J, Lockshin A. Pain perception and nonsuicidal self-injury: a laboratory investigation. Personal Disord. 2010;1(3):170-9.

253. Glenn JJ, Michel BD, Franklin JC, Hooley JM, Nock MK. Pain analgesia among adolescent self-injurers. Psychiatry Res. 2014;220(3):921-6.

254. Gratz KL, Hepworth C, Tull MT, Paulson A, Clarke S, Remington B, et al. An experimental investigation of emotional willingness and physical pain tolerance in deliberate self-harm: the moderating role of interpersonal distress. Compr Psychiatry. 2011;52(1):63-74.

255. Fields HL. Understanding how opioids contribute to reward and analgesia. Reg Anesth Pain Med. 2007;32(3):242-6.

256. Van Ree JM, Niesink RJ, Van Wolfswinkel L, Ramsey NF, Kornet MM, Van Furth WR, *et al.* Endogenous opioids and reward. Eur J Pharmacol. 2000;405(1-3):89-101.

257. Franklin JC, Aaron RV, Arthur MS, Shorkey SP, Prinstein MJ. Nonsuicidal self-injury and diminished pain perception: the role of emotion dysregulation. Compr Psychiatry. 2012;53(6):691-700.

258. Oumaya M, Friedman S, Pham A, Abou Abdallah T, Guelfi JD, Rouillon F. [Borderline personality disorder, self-mutilation and suicide: literature review]. Encephale. 2008;34(5):452-8.

259. Joyce PR, Light KJ, Rowe SL, Cloninger CR, Kennedy MA. Self-mutilation and suicide attempts: relationships to bipolar disorder, borderline personality disorder, temperament and character. Aust N Z J Psychiatry. 2010;44(3):250-7.

260. Kemperman I, Russ MJ, Clark WC, Kakuma T, Zanine E, Harrison K. Pain assessment in self-injurious patients with borderline personality disorder using signal detection theory. Psychiatry Res. 1997;70(3):175-83.

261. Schmahl C, Bohus M, Esposito F, Treede RD, Di Salle F, Greffrath W, et al. Neural correlates of antinociception in borderline personality disorder. Arch Gen Psychiatry. 2006;63(6):659-67.

262. Ludäscher P, Greffrath W, Schmahl C, Kleindienst N, Kraus A, Baumgärtner U, *et al.* A cross-sectional investigation of discontinuation of self-injury and normalizing pain perception in patients with borderline personality disorder. Acta Psychiatr Scand. 2009;120(1):62-70.

263. Kirtley OJ, O'Carroll RE, O'Connor RC. The role of endogenous opioids in non-suicidal self-injurious behavior: methodological challenges. Neurosci Biobehav Rev. 2015;48:186-9.

264. Furczyk K, Schutová B, Michel TM, Thome J, Büttner A. The neurobiology of suicide - A Review of post-mortem studies. J Mol Psychiatry. 2013;1(1):2.

265. Daniel PB, Walker WH, Habener JF. Cyclic AMP signaling and gene regulation. Annu Rev Nutr. 1998;18:353-83.

266. Odagaki Y, García-Sevilla JA, Huguelet P, La Harpe R, Koyama T, Guimón J. Cyclic AMP-mediated signaling components are upregulated in the prefrontal cortex of depressed suicide victims. Brain Res. 2001;898(2):224-31.

267. Ren X, Dwivedi Y, Mondal AC, Pandey GN. Cyclic-AMP response element binding protein (CREB) in the neutrophils of depressed patients. Psychiatry Res. 2011;185(1-2):108-12.

268. Dwivedi Y, Conley RR, Roberts RC, Tamminga CA, Pandey GN. [(3)H]cAMP binding sites and protein kinase a activity in the prefrontal cortex of suicide victims. Am J Psychiatry. 2002;159(1):66-73.

269. Dwivedi Y, Rizavi HS, Shukla PK, Lyons J, Faludi G, Palkovits M, et al. Protein kinase A in postmortem brain of depressed suicide victims: altered expression of specific regulatory and catalytic subunits. Biol Psychiatry. 2004;55(3):234-43.

270. Dwivedi Y, Rao JS, Rizavi HS, Kotowski J, Conley RR, Roberts RC, et al. Abnormal expression and functional characteristics of cyclic adenosine monophosphate response element binding protein in postmortem brain of suicide subjects. Arch Gen Psychiatry. 2003;60(3):273-82.

271. Pandey GN, Dwivedi Y, Ren X, Rizavi HS, Mondal AC, Shukla PK, et al. Brain region specific alterations in the protein and mRNA levels of protein kinase A subunits in the post-mortem brain of teenage suicide victims. Neuropsychopharmacology. 2005;30(8):1548-56.

272. Pandey GN, Dwivedi Y, Ren X, Rizavi HS, Roberts RC, Conley RR. Cyclic AMP response element-binding protein in post-mortem brain of teenage suicide victims: specific decrease in the prefrontal cortex but not the hippocampus. Int J Neuropsychopharmacol. 2007; 10(5):621-9.

273. Dwivedi Y, Pandey GN. Elucidating biological risk factors in suicide: role of protein kinase A. Prog Neuropsychopharmacol Biol Psychiatry. 2011;35(4):831-41.

274. O'Donovan A, Rush G, Hoatam G, Hughes BM, McCrohan A, Kelleher C, *et al*. Suicidal ideation is associated with elevated inflammation in patients with major depressive disorder. Depress Anxiety. 2013;30(4):307-14.

275. Serafini G, Pompili M, Elena Seretti M, Stefani H, Palermo M, Coryell W, *et al*. The role of inflammatory cytokines in suicidal behavior: a systematic review. Eur Neuropsychopharmacol. 2013;23(12):1672-86.

276. Miná VA, Lacerda-Pinheiro SF, Maia LC, Pinheiro RF, Meireles CB, de Souza SI, *et al*. The influence of inflammatory cytokines in physiopathology of suicidal behavior. J Affect Disord. 2014;172C:219-30.

277. van Heeringen C, Bijttebier S, Godfrin K. Suicidal brains: a review of functional and structural brain studies in association with suicidal behaviour. Neurosci Biobehav Rev. 2011;35(3):688-98.

278. van Heeringen K, Bijttebier S, Desmyter S, Vervaet M, Baeken C. Is there a neuroanatomical basis of the vulnerability to suicidal behavior? A coordinate-based meta-analysis of structural and functional MRI studies. Front Hum Neurosci. 2014;8:824.

279. Cox Lippard ET, Johnston JA, Blumberg HP. Neurobiological risk factors for suicide: insights from brain imaging. Am J Prev Med. 2014;47(3 Suppl 2):S152-62.

280. Wallis JD. Orbitofrontal cortex and its contribution to decision-making. Annu Rev Neurosci. 2007;30:31-56.

281. Krawczyk DC. Contributions of the prefrontal cortex to the neural basis of human decision making. Neurosci Biobehav Rev. 2002;26(6):631-64.

282. Carroll R, Metcalfe C, Gunnell D. Hospital presenting self-harm and risk of fatal and non-fatal repetition: systematic review and meta-analysis. PLoS One. 2014;9(2):e89944.

283. Gairin I, House A, Owens D. Attendance at the accident and emergency department in the year before suicide: retrospective study. Br J Psychiatry. 2003;183:28-33.

284. Ness J, Hawton K, Bergen H, Cooper J, Steeg S, Kapur N, *et al.* Alcohol use and misuse, self-harm and subsequent mortality: an epidemiological and longitudinal study from the multicentre study of self-harm in England. Emerg Med J. 2015.

285. Hawton K, Saunders K, Topiwala A, Haw C. Psychiatric disorders in patients presenting to hospital following self-harm: a systematic review. J Affect Disord. 2013;151(3):821-30.

286. Bohanna I, Wang X. Media guidelines for the responsible reporting of suicide: a review of effectiveness. Crisis. 2012;33(4):190-8.

287. Isaac M, Elias B, Katz LY, Belik SL, Deane FP, Enns MW, *et al.* Gatekeeper training as a preventative intervention for suicide: a systematic review. Can J Psychiatry. 2009;54(4):260-8.

288. Sakamoto S, Tanaka E, Kameyama A, Takizawa T, Takizawa S, Fujishima S, *et al.* The effects of suicide prevention measures reported through a psychoeducational video: a practice in Japan. Int J Soc Psychiatry. 2014;60(8):751-8.

289. Sarchiapone M, Mandelli L, Iosue M, Andrisano C, Roy A. Controlling access to suicide means. Int J Environ Res Public Health. 2011;8(12):4550-62.

290. Florentine JB, Crane C. Suicide prevention by limiting access to methods: a review of theory and practice. Soc Sci Med. 2010;70(10): 1626-32.

291. Wood A, Trainor G, Rothwell J, Moore A, Harrington R. Randomized trial of group therapy for repeated deliberate self-harm in adolescents. J Am Acad Child Adolesc Psychiatry. 2001;40(11): 1246-53.

292. Hazell PL, Martin G, McGill K, Kay T, Wood A, Trainor G, *et al.* Group therapy for repeated deliberate self-harm in adolescents: failure of replication of a randomized trial. J Am Acad Child Adolesc Psychiatry. 2009;48(6):662-70.

293. Green JM, Wood AJ, Kerfoot MJ, Trainor G, Roberts C, Rothwell J, *et al.* Group therapy for adolescents with repeated self harm: randomised controlled trial with economic evaluation. BMJ. 2011;342:d682.

294. Huey SJ, Henggeler SW, Rowland MD, Halliday-Boykins CA, Cunningham PB, Pickrel SG, et al. Multisystemic therapy effects on attempted suicide by youths presenting psychiatric emergencies. J Am Acad Child Adolesc Psychiatry. 2004;43(2):183-90.

295. Huey SJ, Henggeler SW, Rowland MD, Halliday-Boykins CA, Cunningham PB, Pickrel SG. Predictors of treatment response for suicidal youth referred for emergency psychiatric hospitalization. J Clin Child Adolesc Psychol. 2005;34(3):582-9.

296. Harrington R, Kerfoot M, Dyer E, McNiven F, Gill J, Harrington V, et al. Randomized trial of a home-based family intervention for children who have deliberately poisoned themselves. J Am Acad Child Adolesc Psychiatry. 1998;37(5):512-8.

297. Harrington R, Kerfoot M, Dyer E, Mcniven F, Gill J, Harrington V, et al. Deliberate self-poisoning in adolescence: why does a brief family intervention work in some cases and not others? J Adolesc. 2000;23(1):13-20.

298. Byford S, Harrington R, Torgerson D, Kerfoot M, Dyer E, Harrington V, et al. Cost-effectiveness analysis of a home-based social work intervention for children and adolescents who have deliberately poisoned themselves. Results of a randomised controlled trial. Br J Psychiatry. 1999;174:56-62.

299. King CA, Klaus N, Kramer A, Venkataraman S, Quinlan P, Gillespie B. The Youth-Nominated Support Team-Version II for suicidal adolescents: A randomized controlled intervention trial. J Consult Clin Psychol. 2009;77(5):880-93.

300. King CA, Kramer A, Preuss L, Kerr DC, Weisse L, Venkataraman S. Youth-Nominated Support Team for Suicidal Adolescents (Version 1): a randomized controlled trial. J Consult Clin Psychol. 2006;74(1):199-206.

301. Chapman AL. Dialectical behavior therapy: current indications and unique elements. Psychiatry (Edgmont). 2006;3(9):62-8.

302. Rathus JH, Miller AL. Dialectical behavior therapy adapted for suicidal adolescents. Suicide Life Threat Behav. 2002;32(2):146-57.

303. Rathus J, Campbell B, Miller A, Smith H. Treatment Acceptability Study of Walking The Middle Path, a New DBT Skills Module for Adolescents and their Families. Am J Psychother. 2015;69(2):163-78.

304. Courtney DB, Flament MF. Adapted Dialectical Behavior Therapy for Adolescents with Self-injurious Thoughts and Behaviors. J Nerv Ment Dis. 2015;203(7):537-44.

305. Fleischhaker C, Munz M, Böhme R, Sixt B, Schulz E. [Dialectical Behaviour Therapy for adolescents (DBT-A)--a pilot study on the therapy of suicidal, parasuicidal, and self-injurious behaviour in female patients with a borderline disorder]. Z Kinder Jugendpsychiatr Psychother. 2006;34(1):15-25; quiz 6-7.

306. Fleischhaker C, Böhme R, Sixt B, Brück C, Schneider C, Schulz E. Dialectical Behavioral Therapy for Adolescents (DBT-A): a clinical Trial for Patients with suicidal and self-injurious Behavior and Borderline Symptoms with a one-year Follow-up. Child Adolesc Psychiatry Ment Health. 2011;5(1):3.

307. Cooney E, Health NZMo, Nui TPotW. Feasibility of Evaluating DBT for Self-harming Adolescents: A Small Randomised Controlled Trial: Te Pou o Te Whakaaro Nui =The National Centre of Mental Health Research and Workforce Development; 2010.

308. Tørmoen AJ, Grøholt B, Haga E, Brager-Larsen A, Miller A, Walby F, et al. Feasibility of dialectical behavior therapy with suicidal and self-harming adolescents with multi-problems: training, adherence, and retention. Arch Suicide Res. 2014;18(4):432-44.

309. Mehlum L, Tørmoen AJ, Ramberg M, Haga E, Diep LM, Laberg S, et al. Dialectical behavior therapy for adolescents with repeated suicidal and self-harming behavior: a randomized trial. J Am Acad Child Adolesc Psychiatry. 2014;53(10):1082-91.

310. Geddes K, Dziurawiec S, Lee CW. Dialectical Behaviour Therapy for the Treatment of Emotion Dysregulation and Trauma Symptoms in Self-Injurious and Suicidal Adolescent Females: A Pilot Programme within a Community-Based Child and Adolescent Mental Health Service. Psychiatry J. 2013;2013:145219.

311. Turner BJ, Austin SB, Chapman AL. Treating nonsuicidal self-injury: a systematic review of psychological and pharmacological interventions. Can J Psychiatry. 2014;59(11):576-85.

312. Linehan MM, Korslund KE, Harned MS, Gallop RJ, Lungu A, Neacsiu AD, *et al.* Dialectical behavior therapy for high suicide risk in individuals with borderline personality disorder: a randomized clinical trial and component analysis. JAMA Psychiatry. 2015;72(5): 475-82.

313. Linehan MM, Comtois KA, Murray AM, Brown MZ, Gallop RJ, Heard HL, *et al.* Two-year randomized controlled trial and follow-up of dialectical behavior therapy vs therapy by experts for suicidal behaviors and borderline personality disorder. Arch Gen Psychiatry. 2006;63(7):757-66.

314. Pistorello J, Fruzzetti AE, Maclane C, Gallop R, Iverson KM. Dialectical behavior therapy (DBT) applied to college students: a randomized clinical trial. J Consult Clin Psychol. 2012;80(6):982-94.

315. Linehan MM, McDavid JD, Brown MZ, Sayrs JH, Gallop RJ. Olanzapine plus dialectical behavior therapy for women with high irritability who meet criteria for borderline personality disorder: a double-blind, placebo-controlled pilot study. J Clin Psychiatry. 2008; 69(6):999-1005.

316. Gibson J, Booth R, Davenport J, Keogh K, Owens T. Dialectical behaviour therapy-informed skills training for deliberate self-harm: a controlled trial with 3-month follow-up data. Behav Res Ther. 2014;60:8-14.

317. (CADTH) CAfDaTiH. Dialectical behaviour therapy in adolescents for suicide prevention: systematic review of clinical-effectiveness. CADTH Technol Overv. 2010;1(1):e0104.

318. Katz LY, Cox BJ, Gunasekara S, Miller AL. Feasibility of dialectical behavior therapy for suicidal adolescent inpatients. J Am Acad Child Adolesc Psychiatry. 2004;43(3):276-82.

319. Markowitz JC, Weissman MM. Interpersonal psychotherapy: principles and applications. World Psychiatry. 2004;3(3):136-9.

320. Zhou X, Hetrick SE, Cuijpers P, Qin B, Barth J, Whittington CJ, *et al.* Comparative efficacy and acceptability of psychotherapies for depression in children and adolescents: A systematic review and network meta-analysis. World Psychiatry. 2015;14(2):207-22.

321. Mufson L, Dorta KP, Wickramaratne P, Nomura Y, Olfson M, Weissman MM. A randomized effectiveness trial of interpersonal psychotherapy for depressed adolescents. Arch Gen Psychiatry. 2004;61(6): 577-84.

322. Mufson L, Yanes-Lukin P, Anderson G. A pilot study of Brief IPT-A delivered in primary care. Gen Hosp Psychiatry. 2015.

323. Tang TC, Jou SH, Ko CH, Huang SY, Yen CF. Randomized study of school-based intensive interpersonal psychotherapy for depressed adolescents with suicidal risk and parasuicide behaviors. Psychiatry Clin Neurosci. 2009;63(4):463-70.

324. David-Ferdon C, Kaslow NJ. Evidence-based psychosocial treatments for child and adolescent depression. J Clin Child Adolesc Psychol. 2008;37(1):62-104.

325. Spirito A, Esposito-Smythers C, Wolff J, Uhl K. Cognitive-behavioral therapy for adolescent depression and suicidality. Child Adolesc Psychiatr Clin N Am. 2011;20(2):191-204.

326. Power PJ, Bell RJ, Mills R, Herrman-Doig T, Davern M, Henry L, *et al.* Suicide prevention in first episode psychosis: the development of a randomised controlled trial of cognitive therapy for acutely suicidal patients with early psychosis. Aust N Z J Psychiatry. 2003; 37(4):414-20.

327. March JS, Silva S, Petrycki S, Curry J, Wells K, Fairbank J, *et al.* The Treatment for Adolescents With Depression Study (TADS): long-term effectiveness and safety outcomes. Arch Gen Psychiatry. 2007;64(10):1132-43.

328. Goodyer IM, Dubicka B, Wilkinson P, Kelvin R, Roberts C, Byford S, *et al.* A randomised controlled trial of cognitive behaviour therapy in adolescents with major depression treated by selective serotonin reuptake inhibitors. The ADAPT trial. Health Technol Assess. 2008;12(14):iii-iv, ix-60.

329. Wilkinson P, Kelvin R, Roberts C, Dubicka B, Goodyer I. Clinical and psychosocial predictors of suicide attempts and nonsuicidal self-injury in the Adolescent Depression Antidepressants and Psycho-therapy Trial (ADAPT). Am J Psychiatry. 2011;168(5):495-501.

330. Emslie GJ, Mayes T, Porta G, Vitiello B, Clarke G, Wagner KD, et al. Treatment of Resistant Depression in Adolescents (TORDIA): week 24 outcomes. Am J Psychiatry. 2010;167(7):782-91.

331. Brent D, Emslie G, Clarke G, Wagner KD, Asarnow JR, Keller M, et al. Switching to another SSRI or to venlafaxine with or without cognitive behavioral therapy for adolescents with SSRI-resistant depression: the TORDIA randomized controlled trial. JAMA. 2008;299(8):901-13.

332. Tarrier N, Taylor K, Gooding P. Cognitive-behavioral interventions to reduce suicide behavior: a systematic review and meta-analysis. Behav Modif. 2008;32(1):77-108.

333. Evans K, Tyrer P, Catalan J, Schmidt U, Davidson K, Dent J, et al. Manual-assisted cognitive-behaviour therapy (MACT): a random-ized controlled trial of a brief intervention with bibliotherapy in the treatment of recurrent deliberate self-harm. Psychol Med. 1999;29(1):19-25.

334. Tyrer P, Thompson S, Schmidt U, Jones V, Knapp M, Davidson K, et al. Randomized controlled trial of brief cognitive behaviour therapy versus treatment as usual in recurrent deliberate self-harm: the POPMACT study. Psychol Med. 2003;33(6):969-76.

335. Weinberg I, Gunderson JG, Hennen J, Cutter CJ. Manual assisted cognitive treatment for deliberate self-harm in borderline personality disorder patients. J Pers Disord. 2006;20(5):482-92.

336. Davidson KM, Brown TM, James V, Kirk J, Richardson J. Manual-assisted cognitive therapy for self-harm in personality disorder and substance misuse: a feasibility trial. Psychiatr Bull (2014). 2014;38(3):108-11.

337. Esposito-Smythers C, Spirito A, Uth R, LaChance H. Cognitive behavioral treatment for suicidal alcohol abusing adolescents: development and pilot testing. Am J Addict. 2006;15 Suppl 1:126-30.

338.   Esposito-Smythers C, Spirito A, Kahler CW, Hunt J, Monti P. Treatment of co-occurring substance abuse and suicidality among adolescents: a randomized trial. J Consult Clin Psychol. 2011; 79(6):728-39.

339.   Richardson T, Stallard P, Velleman S. Computerised cognitive behavioural therapy for the prevention and treatment of depression and anxiety in children and adolescents: a systematic review. Clin Child Fam Psychol Rev. 2010;13(3):275-90.

340.   Rees CS, Hasking P, Breen LJ, Lipp OV, Mamotte C. Group mindfulness based cognitive therapy vs group support for self-injury among young people: study protocol for a randomised controlled trial. BMC Psychiatry. 2015;15:154.

341.   Asarnow JR, Berk M, Hughes JL, Anderson NL. The SAFETY Program: a treatment-development trial of a cognitive-behavioral family treatment for adolescent suicide attempters. J Clin Child Adolesc Psychol. 2015;44(1):194-203.

342.   Ballard ED, Tingey L, Lee A, Suttle R, Barlow A, Cwik M. Emergency department utilization among American Indian adolescents who made a suicide attempt: a screening opportunity. J Adolesc Health. 2014;54(3):357-9.

343.   Rotheram-Borus MJ, Piacentini J, Van Rossem R, Graae F, Cantwell C, Castro-Blanco D, et al. Enhancing treatment adherence with a specialized emergency room program for adolescent suicide attempters. J Am Acad Child Adolesc Psychiatry. 1996;35(5):654-63.

344.   Rotheram-Borus MJ, Piacentini J, Cantwell C, Belin TR, Song J. The 18-month impact of an emergency room intervention for adolescent female suicide attempters. J Consult Clin Psychol. 2000;68(6):1081-93.

345.   Hughes JL, Asarnow JR. Enhanced Mental Health Interventions in the Emergency Department: Suicide and Suicide Attempt Prevention in the ED. Clin Pediatr Emerg Med. 2013;14(1):28-34.

346.   Ougrin D, Zundel T, Ng A, Banarsee R, Bottle A, Taylor E. Trial of Therapeutic Assessment in London: randomised controlled trial of Therapeutic Assessment versus standard psychosocial assessment in

adolescents presenting with self-harm. Arch Dis Child. 2011; 96(2):148-53.

347. Ougrin D, Boege I, Stahl D, Banarsee R, Taylor E. Randomised controlled trial of therapeutic assessment versus usual assessment in adolescents with self-harm: 2-year follow-up. Arch Dis Child. 2013;98(10):772-6.

348. Grupp-Phelan J, McGuire L, Husky MM, Olfson M. A randomized controlled trial to engage in care of adolescent emergency department patients with mental health problems that increase suicide risk. Pediatr Emerg Care. 2012;28(12):1263-8.

349. Smith BD. Self-mutilation and pharmacotherapy. Psychiatry (Edgmont). 2005;2(10):28-37.

350. Ougrin D, Tranah T, Stahl D, Moran P, Asarnow JR. Therapeutic interventions for suicide attempts and self-harm in adolescents: systematic review and meta-analysis. J Am Acad Child Adolesc Psychiatry. 2015;54(2):97-107.e2.

351. Hawton K, Witt KG, Taylor Salisbury TL, Arensman E, Gunnell D, Hazell P, et al. Pharmacological interventions for self-harm in adults. Cochrane Database Syst Rev. 2015;7:CD011777.

352. Nickel MK, Muehlbacher M, Nickel C, Kettler C, Pedrosa Gil F, Bachler E, et al. Aripiprazole in the treatment of patients with borderline personality disorder: a double-blind, placebo-controlled study. Am J Psychiatry. 2006;163(5):833-8.

353. Nickel MK, Loew TH, Pedrosa Gil F. Aripiprazole in treatment of borderline patients, part II: an 18-month follow-up. Psychopharmacology (Berl). 2007;191(4):1023-6.

354. Stone M, Laughren T, Jones ML, Levenson M, Holland PC, Hughes A, et al. Risk of suicidality in clinical trials of antidepressants in adults: analysis of proprietary data submitted to US Food and Drug Administration. BMJ. 2009;339:b2880.

355. Tandt H, Audenaert K, van Heeringen C. [SSRIs (selective serotonin reuptake inhibitors) and suicidality in adults, adolescents and children]. Tijdschr Psychiatr. 2009;51(6):387-93.

356. Dudley M, Goldney R, Hadzi-Pavlovic D. Are adolescents dying by suicide taking SSRI antidepressants? A review of observational studies. Australas Psychiatry. 2010;18(3):242-5.

357. Valuck RJ, Libby AM, Sills MR, Giese AA, Allen RR. Antidepressant treatment and risk of suicide attempt by adolescents with major depressive disorder: a propensity-adjusted retrospective cohort study. CNS Drugs. 2004;18(15):1119-32.

358. Hassanin H, Harbi A, Saif A, Davis J, Easa D, Harrigan R. Changes in antidepressant medications prescribing trends in children and adolescents in Hawai'i following the FDA black box warning. Hawaii Med J. 2010;69(1):17-9.

359. Libby AM, Brent DA, Morrato EH, Orton HD, Allen R, Valuck RJ. Decline in treatment of pediatric depression after FDA advisory on risk of suicidality with SSRIs. Am J Psychiatry. 2007;164(6):884-91.

360. Libby AM, Orton HD, Valuck RJ. Persisting decline in depression treatment after FDA warnings. Arch Gen Psychiatry. 2009;66(6):633-9.

361. Lu CY, Zhang F, Lakoma MD, Madden JM, Rusinak D, Penfold RB, et al. Changes in antidepressant use by young people and suicidal behavior after FDA warnings and media coverage: quasi-experimental study. BMJ. 2014;348:g3596.

362. Olfson M, Schoenbaum M. Link between FDA antidepressant warnings and increased suicide attempts in young people is questionable. BMJ. 2014;349:g5614.

363. Barber C, Azrael D, Miller M. Study findings on FDA antidepressant warnings and suicide attempts in young people: a false alarm? BMJ. 2014;349:g5645.

364. Bartlett RO. Proxy for suicide attempts was inappropriate in study of changes in antidepressant use after FDA warnings. BMJ. 2014;349:g5644.

365. Nardo JM. Impossible to draw meaningful conclusions from study of changes in antidepressant use after FDA warnings. BMJ. 2014;349:g5643.

366. Gøtzsche PC. Study of study of changes in antidepressant use after FDA warnings is not reliable. BMJ. 2014;349:g5623.

367. Miller M, Pate V, Swanson SA, Azrael D, White A, Stürmer T. Antidepressant class, age, and the risk of deliberate self-harm: a propensity score matched cohort study of SSRI and SNRI users in the USA. CNS Drugs. 2014;28(1):79-88.

368. Coupland C, Hill T, Morriss R, Arthur A, Moore M, Hippisley-Cox J. Antidepressant use and risk of suicide and attempted suicide or self harm in people aged 20 to 64: cohort study using a primary care database. BMJ. 2015;350:h517.

369. Didham RC, McConnell DW, Blair HJ, Reith DM. Suicide and self-harm following prescription of SSRIs and other antidepressants: confounding by indication. Br J Clin Pharmacol. 2005;60(5):519-25.

370. Spirito A, Plummer B, Gispert M, Levy S, Kurkjian J, Lewander W, et al. Adolescent suicide attempts: outcomes at follow-up. Am J Orthopsychiatry. 1992;62(3):464-8.

371. Trautman PD, Stewart N, Morishima A. Are adolescent suicide attempters noncompliant with outpatient care? J Am Acad Child Adolesc Psychiatry. 1993;32(1):89-94.

372. Groholt B, Ekeberg O. Prognosis after adolescent suicide attempt: mental health, psychiatric treatment, and suicide attempts in a nine-year follow-up study. Suicide Life Threat Behav. 2009;39(2):125-36.

373. Piacentini J, Rotheram-Borus MJ, Gillis JR, Graae F, Trautman P, Cantwell C, et al. Demographic predictors of treatment attendance among adolescent suicide attempters. J Consult Clin Psychol. 1995;63(3):469-73.

374. Votta E, Manion I. Suicide, high-risk behaviors, and coping style in homeless adolescent males' adjustment. J Adolesc Health. 2004;34(3):237-43.

375. Taylor EA, Stansfeld SA. Children who poison themselves. II. Prediction of attendance for treatment. Br J Psychiatry. 1984;145:132-5.

376. Burns CD, Cortell R, Wagner BM. Treatment compliance in adolescents after attempted suicide: a 2-year follow-up study. J Am Acad Child Adolesc Psychiatry. 2008;47(8):948-57.

377. Spirito A, Lewander WJ, Levy S, Kurkjian J, Fritz G. Emergency department assessment of adolescent suicide attempters: factors related to short-term follow-up outcome. Pediatr Emerg Care. 1994;10(1):6-12.

378. Granboulan V, Roudot-Thoraval F, Lemerle S, Alvin P. Predictive factors of post-discharge follow-up care among adolescent suicide attempters. Acta Psychiatr Scand. 2001;104(1):31-6.

379. Ougrin D, Latif S. Specific psychological treatment versus treatment as usual in adolescents with self-harm: systematic review and meta-analysis. Crisis. 2011;32(2):74-80.

380. Yuan SNVK, Ka Ho Robin.Ougrin, Dennis. Treatment Engagement in Specific Psychological Treatment Versus Treatment as Usual for Self-Harm Adolescents: Systematic Review and Meta-Analysis. Unpublished; 2015.

381. Pitman A. Policy on the prevention of suicidal behaviour; one treatment for all may be an unrealistic expectation. J R Soc Med. 2007;100(10):461-4.

382. Sareen J, Isaak C, Katz LY, Bolton J, Enns MW, Stein MB. Promising strategies for advancement in knowledge of suicide risk factors and prevention. Am J Prev Med. 2014;47(3 Suppl 2):S257-63.

383. Bridge JA, Horowitz LM, Fontanella CA, Grupp-Phelan J, Campo JV. Prioritizing research to reduce youth suicide and suicidal behavior. Am J Prev Med. 2014;47(3 Suppl 2):S229-34.

384. Wyman PA. Developmental approach to prevent adolescent suicides: research pathways to effective upstream preventive interventions. Am J Prev Med. 2014;47(3 Suppl 2):S251-6.

www.ingramcontent.com/pod-product-compliance
Lightning Source LLC
Chambersburg PA
CBHW072000220326

41599CB00034BA/7060